MISADVENTURE

LESSONS LEARNED FROM A LIFE OF UPS & DOWNS

Hardback edition published in the UK July 2021 by FBS Publishing Ltd.
This edition published October 2021.
68 The Street, Attleborough, Norfolk NR17 1TP
ISBN 978-1-7398358-1-1

Text Edited by Alasdair McKenzie

DEDICATION

For Doug.
Thank you for the inspiration to believe
and for showing the way.

By the same author:

Everest: It's Not About the Summit

MISADVENTURE
LESSONS LEARNED FROM A LIFE OF UPS & DOWNS

Ellis J Stewart

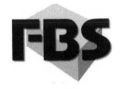

Fabulous BookS
www.fbs-publishing.co.uk

CONTENTS

WE BECAME MOUNTAINS
Anthony Frobisher

I stared into the abyss,
Crevasse drawn.
A beckoning darkness.
A cold embrace.
The hidden sun,
A lost warmth.

My face scarred, wearing
A carapace of sadness,
Solid, frozen, immovable.
My limbs numb, pained.
The ache of wounds
Sustained long before.

I wearied, afraid to fall,
Sapped and drained of will by
The punishing cold, unforgiving.
I could not go on, let me fall.
Let me surrender to cold and darkness.
Let me fall, let me fall.

A hand reached out,
Pulled me from the abyss.
Chiselled the sorrow from
My face, and rescued
A forgotten smile.
Let's climb he said.

We brothers held the rope
Of kinship and friendship,
Climbing together as one.
Our summits reached,
Each personal, different.
Yet we shared the same view.

Where friendship conquers
Fear and sadness and loss.
Where warmth of kindness spreads
Like sunrise and no cold penetrates.
Where we will never fall,
Secured, tethered to friendship.

I climbed, I failed.
But when we climbed
We succeeded.
I climbed and
was nothing.
But when
we climbed,
We became
mountains.

FOREWORD

BY ROB 'ZED' METCALFE

As I sat on the bench in my mum's front garden on a cold and sunny February day, holding a copy of a book I was reading about an attempt on Mount Everest, little did I realise that just two weeks later I would be sitting on the same bench talking in person to the author of that book.

I had always had a deep fascination when it came to Everest, ever since I was young. I had always dreamed that one day I would stand on top of the world's highest mountain. But in 2018, my world came crashing down around me when I was diagnosed with Synovial Sarcoma, a rare form of soft tissue cancer. In March 2019 I was told that I was terminally ill, and my life was going to be cut short considerably by this disease. My dream of going to Mount Everest, let alone standing on the summit, was now always going to remain a dream.

Two weeks before that appointment in March, I met Ellis, after he had driven down from his hometown in the North East specially to see me. Me! Just an everyday chap who likes to walk up hills and had a big dream of summiting Everest.

We talked about lots of things that day, Everest, life, and the future. Before he left, he gave me a signed copy of his book. From that day forward we became great friends, and I have experienced moments in my life with Ellis since then that I will never forget.

The adventure, or should I say the misadventure, through this beautiful thing called life is to be cherished, enjoyed and revelled in.

No matter the setbacks or the hardships that Ellis has faced, whether it be on the side of Mount Everest or in his everyday life, he is one of the kindest, most caring and truest-to-his-heart men that I have had the pleasure of knowing. He is focused and determined to keep his dreams alive, not only in the mountains but in his home life.

Mountains, like life, have ascents and descents, climbs and abseils, and they do not always go to plan. With a technical climb, if you do not use protection and ropes, one of three things will happen; either you won't climb because it's too difficult, you climb and fall, or you climb and succeed. And abseiling without a rope ... well, that is just falling. Making the right decisions in the mountains is crucial, and usually your life depends on your decision-making skills.

Luckily, life, unlike mountains, can be more forgiving. The consequences of the decisions made and those moments that are completely out of your control, like abseiling without a rope (falling), are all part of the misadventure of life. It is how you pick yourself back up and start the ascent again that counts.

Back to the bench that day. I sat fixated, post-cancer diagnosis, turning the pages of Ellis's book about not reaching the summit of the world's highest mountain, twice, and getting an insight into how an everyday chap deals with everyday life while dreaming big. I had the sudden realisation that the misadventures are all part of the adventure. As Ellis himself said, the summit is less important than the overall journey.

Ellis has inspired me, and many others who have had their dreams broken, to keep on dreaming, keep on striving, thriving and making our misadventures part of the adventure of life. And for that, I will always be forever grateful to him.

Rob 'Zed' Metcalfe. November 2020.

PROLOGUE

I wanted to die. Of that I was certain. Nothing mattered anymore. All that I could focus on was what I was going to do that morning.

I was a failure in every sense of the word. I had not been able to look at myself in a mirror and be happy with what I saw staring back for a very long time. I despised myself and my existence. The voice inside my head had won. I had given in and accepted my fate.

'Well, you have really messed things up this time, Ellis. Do it. End this suffering. No one will miss you anyway, you waste of space.'

I was living in hell, except my hell only existed in my head. My brain was trying to make sense of all the messages I was struggling desperately to understand. But as much as I tried to make sense of the darkness that was swirling through my mind, I couldn't. I was too weak to fight anymore.

I sat in my home office, staring at the pictures of Mount Everest that adorned the walls. Tibetan prayer flags hung down from the ceiling, fluttering gently with the heat from the radiator.

I stared at a picture of Everest again, this time focusing on the summit. This was a place where I had dared to tread but was denied. I yanked it down from the wall and slammed it on the floor. The glass frame smashed into pieces.

'Come on, Ella, let's go.'

My dog obediently followed, wagging her tail at the prospect of going out for a walk. I bundled her into the boot of the car and drove to a nearby beach, five minutes from my home. This was a beach I would often bring her to for her daily exercise. It was windswept, wild and rugged. The coastline in this part of the country was dramatic and usually desolate. After visiting almost daily, I knew when the beach would be busy, and I knew when it wouldn't. First thing in the morning it was rarely crowded. Maybe one or two other dog walkers, but that was about it.

I parked up and strode down the steep steps onto the beach. There was a stiff breeze blowing. The sand was being picked up by the wind and was drifting menacingly across the beach, making strange patterns as it did. It stung my shins as I continued to walk to the sea.

I could see a few other people off in the distance, a good 500 metres or so away. That was fine, I reasoned. I would have time to do what I had intended before they would reach me.

It was a cold day in November, but not unduly so. I was dressed in shorts, my running trainers, a T-shirt, and a mid-weight down jacket. On my head, I wore a beanie.

At the water's edge, I put my pack down on the sand. I pulled out the bottle of whiskey I had brought. I began to speak to the bottle as I took swig after swig.

'So, this is how it's going to be, eh, Jack? Just you and me.'

I felt the alcohol burning my throat as I poured and gulped.

Ella began to bark. She wanted me to throw a stone so she could retrieve it and bring it back, as was our custom. I picked up a smooth round pebble and threw it as hard as I could. She immediately gave chase. I then strode into the sea.

I could feel the cold water numbing my exposed legs. I walked further into the cold abyss. I wasn't going to stop. The water reached my waist, and then just below my chest. The cold made it impossible to breathe. I gasped for air—not that I wanted it. With my entire body numb, I kept going. Suddenly, the seabed gave way, a few feet. The water went over my shoulders. There was just my head above the waterline now. The voices started to take over again.

'Do it. This will all be over soon.'

Back on the beach, Ella barked relentlessly. I also became vaguely aware of someone shouting.

'Hi, hello. Is everything okay?'

I put my head under the water and felt the icy sharpness of a million swords, all stabbing into my skull at the same time. The noise of the current was deafening.

What the fuck was I doing? How had it come to this? What had I done to deserve this?

I accidentally swallowed a mouth full of seawater and closed my eyes.

INTRODUCTION

'Our bravest and best lessons are not learned through success, but through misadventure.'
Amos Bronson Alcott

I never thought I would write a book. What would I write about? My life hasn't exactly been that noteworthy. Never mind being a Jack of all trades. I am a Jack of no trades, master of none.

But we all have a story to tell. Some of the best stories ever told come from the minds of us normal folk—your next-door neighbour, or an old schoolteacher perhaps; those of us not in the limelight.

Everest gave me my first book. A story of misadventure on the world's highest mountain which I subsequently would go on to write about. I never for one second expected that I would pick up my quill and ink and be audacious enough to think I had another book in me. I mean, again, what would I write about this time? Everest: It's About the Summit?

If I ever did write another book, about a 'successful' climb of the mountain, I have always thought that it would not be as well-received as my previous story of tragedy and disaster on the mountain. Who wants to read about someone climbing a mountain, where he succeeds? Man climbs Everest. The end. In decades gone by, this would have made for a very compelling story, but the mountain is climbed by hundreds of individuals every year now. Not that I am bitter you understand.

I believe the spice of life is in its adversity. Don't get me wrong, I would much rather have climbed the mountain, than live through what did happen. But the disasters on Everest became my story, and I cannot do anything to change that. I embraced it and accepted it had now become part of who I am.

When I recently took a moment to reflect, I realised I did have another story. It had been there all along without me realising it. And it didn't involve a single mountain this time. This story is one we can all write. It is the story of our real lives. The everyday adventures and misadventures that lurk around every corner. Real-life can be far more fascinating. You do not need to visit places such as mountains to experience success or glory, danger, or mishap.

I won't deny it is this danger and mishap that sells books and makes for amazing stories of hardship and resilience. It is no coincidence that the 2015 Hollywood movie *Everest* is about a real-life disaster on Mount Everest where lots of people died. The 1997 blockbuster *Titanic*, one of the highest-grossing movies of all time, is about a real-life disaster where lots of people die. *Impossible*, a film starring Ewan McGregor, about a family who decide to spend Christmas in Thailand is about … you guessed it, a real-life disaster where lots of people die. There is a definite pattern. And it usually involves death.

However, you don't need to be involved in misadventure on such a tragic and disastrous scale for it to leave its mark. Misadventure often can be found in the everyday, mundane details of daily life. It is in the minuscule details which we often overlook. It is within us and around us. It gives us character and strength. It can make us who we are today. But we don't necessarily realise it at the time.

I have previously written about a large-scale misadventure where a lot of people died, and I will skim over that in a later chapter. This book, on the other hand, will focus on the misadventures of normal life—the misfortunate, everyday type of situations and circumstances we can all find ourselves involved in. I think we thrive on the misfortune of life, not because we are all a bit psychotic and love to see misery, but because we love to see the underdog story. We like to read about, watch and admire those who have bounced back, shown resilience and achieved against a backdrop of overwhelming odds.

That's why people bought and read my Everest book, not because they wanted to learn about me. No one knew who I was. My name didn't sell that book, the title did. It drew people in. So, if it's not about the summit, then what is it about? People wanted to read about Mount Everest and the disasters that occurred. I just told the story of those events from my point of view. My back story was just a by-product of the overall Everest misadventure from those two years. This book, on the other hand, offers a glimpse into the seemingly routine and frequent misadventures of my everyday life. This time, it's about me! It offers an exposé of my life since Everest and looks back at some of the more defining moments of my life before. Some of the mishaps and trivialities of my life are laid bare as I take you on a chaotic and often unpredictable journey.

There are lots of little takeaways and lessons that I have learned along the way. Mainly not to be a dipshit in life, but we will deal with that as we go.

In my life, other than my wife and children, I have never experienced any significant wins. The type that would completely turn my life upside down; winning the lottery, for instance, or buying in to an investment that turned gold. I have never inherited a single penny, nor been able to buy a shiny new £100,000 sports car. I have been a dreamer more than an achiever, and I have spent years of my life regretting the things I didn't do rather than what I did. I have run multiple business ventures, but I wouldn't say I've been a success in any of them. Life is a game in which we are all players, and we all have our defined roles to play. I am still in the game, only just, and I am still seeking that first significant win. I guess we all are. No one wants to be a loser in this game of life.

If I had stopped dawdling and procrastinating, I could have written this book much earlier than I did. There are not many things in life that I have perfected to a fine art, but in procrastination, I truly take the crown.

Hopefully, by now, we are on our way to recovery from the coronavirus pandemic that emerged at the end of 2019, causing massive upheaval throughout 2020 and well over three million deaths around the world. Lockdown, quarantine, isolation, social distancing; these are words and phrases that have for evermore had their meanings altered, in ways we will remember for the rest of our days.

It's been six years since I returned home from Everest and four since I wrote about it in my book that was subsequently published. I feel like I have been living my life in lockdown ever since.

At the time I wrote that Everest book, I couldn't find a traditional book publisher interested in my story of woe and peril on the highest mountain in the world. But this didn't stop me, as you will later discover. My book went on to top the Kindle mountaineering chart on Amazon in the UK, several times over.

This is a bit clichéd, but I am going to say it anyway. If you believe in trying to achieve something, then go for it. Don't take no for an answer or let anyone tell you 'no' if you believe strongly in whatever it is.

It's far too easy to be told no and to walk away from something because it seems to be 'too problematic'. There are too many obstacles blocking your way to success. It's 'too difficult'. But aren't obstacles meant to be tackled? And often, head-on. Success is always so much sweeter when the battle for victory was harder in the first place.

If the Formula One star Lewis Hamilton, a boy who grew up on a council estate in Stevenage, can become the greatest driver of all time in a sport dominated by money, it shows that sometimes in life, impossible can become possible. I am not comparing writing and self-publishing a book on the same level as winning seven Formula One World Championships, but the belief is the same. If you believe you can, then maybe you can.

It was not easy getting my Everest story to print, but I never faltered. I stuck to the course, in the same way that I stuck the course with this book. If you are reading or listening to these words, then it's obvious: I was successful again, so well done me. Here, have a glass of champers, Ellis!

As I have said, I think we all have stories to tell. Everyone should write a book at least once in their life. I am always in awe of speaking to people and listening to stories of their respective lives. Humans are intriguing creatures. We are all complex and fascinating. Our stories and life experiences are what define us. They put the meat on the bones of our existence. If not for stories, there would be nothing in life. No movies, no music, no love, and no religions too. Don't worry, I'm not about to break out in a John Lennon song. If Joanne Rowling, an unemployed young mother, had not sat down and started writing that day in a coffee shop in Edinburgh, can you imagine how worse off a world this would be? A world without Harry Potter is not a world I can bring myself to imagine. Damn it, I have broken into a Lennon song again. My point is, stories are the flesh and blood of our lives. We need stories to keep the wheels turning and the world spinning.

Throughout this voyage of life, not all of it will be smooth sailing. We will all, at various points on this voyage, undoubtedly encounter stormy seas and ferocious squalls. In this book, I want to share with you some of these lesser storms I have encountered. Not the huge cataclysmic mountain storms. Been there, done that, wore the T-shirt and wrote the book. I am talking about the ones that at first seem trivial and petty, but when you look back upon them you realise they are the building blocks that shape your life.

Why have I written a book with a title as ambiguous as Misadventure? Quite simply, misadventure is the story of my life. It is the perfect title, to sum up the various encounters and misfortunes of my life. Misadventure and failure go hand in hand within the pages you are about to read. These two terms are not mutually exclusive. My failures in life have often come about because of my many misadventures.

In English Law, misadventure can be defined as death caused by a person accidentally while performing a legal act without negligence or intent to harm. It can also mean an unfortunate incident or mishap. For the sake of transparency, we will go with the second of those meanings for the remainder of the book. My misadventures have not caused anyone's untimely demise—not yet, anyway.

Since I returned home from Mount Everest, my journey has been one of continued self-discovery. But when you think about it, shouldn't every single day of our lives be a journey of discovery and self-learning?

I sometimes feel as though I am still up on that mountain, trying to overcome some insurmountable odds. But odds are there to be overcome, and rule books are designed to be torn up. I discover more about who I am with each passing day.

I have always extolled the virtues of having goals and ambitions in life and then trying to achieve those goals, learning to become resilient along the way. Whether this mindset leads to the achievement of the goal and ultimately leads to a successful life, or leads to one of repeated failure, does not matter. What matters is picking yourself up and dusting yourself down. Again, and again, if you must. It is this ability to recover that is key. If you quit and give up trying, then what's the point in being alive? The minute you stop trying is the minute you start dying. It is important to be able to look at yourself in a mirror and be at ease with what you see staring back. It is so important, in fact, that I am going to repeat it. It is important to be able to look at yourself in a mirror and be happy with what you see.

Why have I emphasized this point twice? Because, as recently as a year ago, I didn't like what I saw when I gazed into a mirror. I had let my failures consume me, instead of letting them become my friend. This lack of self-worth and self-hatred I felt for myself took me down a slippery slope, into a pit of despair, which I was very nearly unable to climb back out of. I am speaking from real-life experience when I say you must learn to love yourself before anyone else can. Recently, that became a huge problem for me. I forgot how to love, like and respect myself. And because of this, I didn't understand why anyone else would, either. I pushed people away, those who were closest to me. I shut them out. I closed down and buried my head in the sand, and it very nearly cost me everything.

This book is not written as a motivational self-help book where I get to show off about how great my life is, and how you too can be like me if you follow these simple steps. Because it should be obvious to you already that my life has not always been—well, quite frankly—that great. Real-life does not follow a conventional path of wisdom.

I don't believe that it's possible to read about how to become motivational. You either are, or you're not, based on the real-life you have lived and the choices you have made. But by reading about real life—in this case, my real life—you can become motivated. Being motivational and motivated is not the same thing. I hope with this book you can become the latter.

There will be certain chapters of this book dedicated to failures I have personally experienced. Failure can floor you, but it needn't keep you down. It only keeps you down if you choose to stay down. It is rising every time and how we rise each time that makes us resilient human beings.

I believe becoming resilient to the effects of failure is the biggest superpower a person can possess. If you can get to a headspace where you become comfortably numb with failure, life suddenly doesn't seem so bad. After all, success is always less funny than failure, and we all need laughter in life.

Thomas Edison is famous for many things, not least for inventing the incandescent light bulb, the phonograph and the motion picture camera. For every successful invention he created, however, he failed with hundreds more. He once said, 'I have not failed, I have just found 10,000 ways that do not work.' Failure is good. Without failure, we cannot grow into the person we perhaps strive to be. Your job in this life is to accept failure as the norm, but don't blame it for being the reason you are not where you want to be. Become more Edison and less yourself.

There are no limits to what can be accomplished once you begin to see failure as your friend. We should all like failure, because it is so easy to achieve. Failure need not define you nor defeat you. You will not fail to reach your goals because you failed once or twice along the way, but you will fail to hit them if you begin to doubt yourself. Never let doubt into your way of thinking. Doubt should be your enemy, not failure.

Failure has been a feature of this life of mine throughout the book you are about to read, so it feels fitting to begin this journey by speaking about it. Some of the most famous people on this planet were, by their definitions, complete failures before they became successful. Think about these four—on the face of it, successful—household names who were not always so graced and blessed.

- Henry Ford—Ford's early businesses failed and left him continually broke before he found eventual success with the Ford Motor Company.

- Walt Disney—In his early life, Disney was fired from a newspaper for lacking imagination. A lot of his earlier businesses met with failure and financial ruin before he found the formula for success.

- Charles Darwin—Gave up on a medical career and was criticised by his father as being bone idle. He was considered as having below-average intelligence at best by his old schoolmasters.

- Oprah Winfrey—Nowadays one of the most successful and richest women on the planet. But it was not always that way. Oprah came from an abusive childhood and was once fired from her job as a TV reporter for being 'unfit for TV'.

You see. There is hope for us all yet.

In your life, you may yourself experience a failure, to some lesser or larger degree. How you bounce back from that failure is what defines you. You either crumble and let the failure consume you, or you get back on your feet and you go again, and again, and again, as long as it takes. The building blocks to a life spent comfortably in your skin begins by analysing the reasons for your failure. I have never failed at anything I have ever done, said no one ever.

I failed at my aims to climb Mount Everest several years ago, but it wasn't my fault. There was nothing I could do to stop an avalanche one year and an earthquake the next. Had I failed in my efforts because I was not fit enough for the challenge, then you could argue my failure was mine to own, caused by not wanting it enough. In my misadventures on the world's highest mountain, there was also an element of being just plain unlucky. I picked the worst years imaginable, one after the other, to attempt to climb the mountain. What was I thinking?

Do we need to experience failure in order to grow and truly appreciate what matters in life? For a lot of us, the answer to this is yes. To discover who we are and what we want out of this life, we should experience a failure to some lesser or larger degree. Whether that failure is not getting the grade you wanted in an exam, or almost dying on the side of a mountain when an earthquake hits, it is all relative to the individual. To the 18-year-old who misses out on a place at Oxford University due to getting one grade less than required, this failure can feel like the end of the world, just as when my Everest dream imploded around me it most definitely felt like the end of my world.

Even if you are happy and content, the one thing you can count on to try and spoil the party will be failure. You might be lucky enough to only experience small failures now and then, such as stumbling over your words whilst giving a work presentation. That's no big deal, at the end of the day. You might have just lost your company a new contract, but so what? No one died. You learn from it; you practise for next time and you do a better job and win a bigger contract. It is a recoverable failure, even if you were fired.

Big failures in life—I mean the huge failures, the type which I have experienced myself—now these are the real testing failures of life. Hopefully, you will never experience a failure of this magnitude. But if you do, it need not break you. It is possible to learn from it and overcome. Spending over 70,000 USD hoping to reach the summit of a mountain and then seeing your hopes crushed two years running; now that is a real crushing failure. Whether that failure was caused by yourself, or—as in my case—was outside of my control, it can have a dramatic and profound knock-on effect for the rest of your life. Failing my exams at school would come back to haunt me 30 years later. Recently failing to secure employment caused me to question my worthiness as a husband and a father.

Failure can be personal, and it can be unique to you. The magnitude of the failure will largely dictate how you react and how you either recover or succumb. Despite everything, I believe we should not take life too seriously! Isn't life serious enough already? Let's face it, none of us are going to get out of it alive, so why be all serious and dramatic? A wise man once said, 'Life is short, smile while you still have teeth.' However, just because I believe we shouldn't take life seriously doesn't mean we shouldn't give a flying fuck. On the contrary, we most definitely should. After all, if you are living your life without giving an 'f', you are only living a lie.

I am 47 now, but I still feel as though I am learning every day from the mistakes I have made, and still do make. Hopefully, I have years left to give to this life to try to correct some of these mistakes.

Money, and the pursuit of attaining lots of it, has never really motivated me. Yes, I know this is an odd thing to say, but it's true. And I guess the reason why it has never motivated me is that I have never really had it. Don't get me wrong, I see all the good things that can come from being financially comfortable. Nice holidays, a nice big flashy car, the latest iPhone or computer, and even another expedition to climb 'that' mountain. However, I am not so sure that we need those things to be happy. Do I need to climb Everest to be deemed a success in life? No. Do I need to do so to be happy? Possibly, but that happiness will be fleeting. Eventually, the euphoria will wear off.

For everyone who read my Everest book, this book is a sequel, a prequel and a book of now. There will be lots of little life lessons, contained within the pages, that I have learned along the way. Each of these experiences has generally coincided with one of my many misadventures. But it is these misadventures that have made me the person I am today.

I don't want you to think my life is one big misadventure and mishap after another. Of course, it isn't. There have been some successes and victories along the way. Can you imagine how rubbish my life would be if I had not prevailed at anything? Ironically, it is these tales of misfortune which eventually led to the successes in my life. I believe that, although not impossible, it is harder to succeed unless you have experienced some form of hardship or failure.

I take nothing for granted and accept that almost anything in this life can happen. Even as I write these words, the United Kingdom is in the grip of a second national lockdown, caused by a global viral pandemic. This is a misadventure on a massive scale which we are all living through. During these uncertain times, I hope this book will provide some comfort, illumination and amusement to all who read it.

I invite you to come along on this journey with me. You had better strap in and hold on tight, though; it's going to get rough and choppy. But I promise you it will be worth it.

Ellis. November 2020

CHAPTER ONE
MY GROWING PAINS

'For in every adult there dwells the child that was,
and in every child, there lies the adult that will be.'
John Connolly

I was an ugly baby. I would never have won any bonnie baby
or cute child competitions. My mum says otherwise, but I
beg to differ. She blames my initial ugliness on the ventouse
(vacuum style medical device) that was used to try to suck
me out of her womb. Now isn't that a lovely image!

From the very beginning, I settled into a childhood of
misadventure and mischief. By the time I was a small boy, I
had spent more time in a hospital than I had at school. I
was also a big baby. I weighed in at a whopping 9lb 14oz.
Ouch! Being a big baby spilt over into being a big three-
year-old and then a big five-year-old, and for a while, there
was grave concern that I was going to keep getting bigger
and bigger. I was also bow-legged, which meant that when I
walked, I looked like I was permanently straddling a horse.
Everywhere I went, people would stare and laugh at this
chubby little blonde boy who looked like the love child of
John Wayne and Humpty Dumpty.

Luckily, the fear that I was heading for a life as Augustus
Gloop by the time I was 10 years old thankfully didn't
materialise, and for a very good reason: I discovered being
outside. Being outside meant I was getting natural exercise,

and plenty of it. I never liked coming home at night when called, and I would frequently skip mealtimes, choosing instead to spend my 12 pence daily pocket money in the corner shop on a mix-up bag of sweets.

The only thing that would get me home in an evening was my mum mentioning The Child Catcher, the villain from the 1968 family musical *Chitty Chitty Bang Bang*. What kind of person puts the most terrifying and villainous character ever created into a family movie? Roald Dahl has a lot to answer for. He completely ruined my childhood. I still get a shudder down my spine if I watch the movie today with my girls—which I try to avoid at all costs, I might add.

I don't recall an awful lot from my secondary school days. I had a mediocre school experience, if I am truthful. I was not a bad student, but then I was not academically gifted either. This was reflected when I left school with one GCSE, in History, to my name.

It was while I was at secondary school that I joined a youth cadet unit, affiliated to the Royal Marines. This changed everything for me. I wanted to be a Royal Marine when I left school. Education no longer mattered. I had it all mapped out. After effectively flunking my education and putting all my effort into signing up for the military, I was left bereft when my worst fears were confirmed. I failed the medical due to hearing loss I had suffered in one ear, caused by infections in my younger years. I enrolled at the local further education college instead to study for a qualification in swimming pool management. I wanted to do a sports science course, but my grades from school, being as abysmal as they were, prevented this. I had to settle for learning about PH, alkaline levels and water chemistry instead.

As I mentioned in my book about Everest, I am not too sure just exactly where my drive to climb the mountain came from, but I think it probably had a lot to do with my love of being outside and my quest for adventure. That, and possibly some of my more mischievous escapades as a youth.

One such caper led to my first full-page newspaper report for climbing. There was an old and dilapidated chapel which had been sat empty in the centre of town. I would often wonder what it would be like inside. What adventures would I find? Would there be a pirate ship full of treasure? I had just recently watched *The Goonies* at the cinema, about a group of misfit kids who discover an ancient map, which leads them on an adventure in which they discover a ship full of treasure. It was an enticing proposition.

To a 12-year-old boy, it presented an exciting adventure one Saturday afternoon. I persuaded a friend of mine at the time that it would be fun if we were to go inside.

'We might even find some treasure.' I said.

He agreed to come.

I stood on my friend's shoulders and was able to reach a window ledge and pull myself up, into a rather imposing auditorium. The floor had completely given way, exposing beams and timbers. Carefully balancing as if walking on a tightrope was the only safe way to move around. I helped my friend in, and we set off exploring the ruins. We somehow climbed our way to the very top of the building and into the loft area, where a gaping hole in the tiles gave access to the chapel roof. As I stood on the very top of the roof that Saturday afternoon, smiling and waving to the photographers below, little did I realise that I was about to grace the front cover of the local newspaper.

The following Monday, underneath the headline 'Lunatic Yobs Risk Their Life in Historic Building Break In,' was a close up of my friend and I with our thumbs up. My mum was mortified. It was so obviously me on the top of the building and now on the front cover of the newspaper.

Besides, the police had already taken me home and given me a stern warning about the dangers of going into old buildings. I remember one of the police officers couldn't stop laughing throughout the whole telling off I got, and he patted me on the head when he left, calling me a wee tyke. I may have been a rascal back then, but I was certainly an adventurous rascal. I did think the headline to the article was a bit harsh. It was never a break in! It was exploration and adventure at its finest, to a 12-year-old boy at least.

**

It was around this time that my family unit had broken down once more, as my mum and stepdad went through a messy divorce. Although I was too young the first time around, when Mum left my biological father, this time I was very aware of what was happening and the consequences this would have on my home life, but most significantly the effect this would have on my mum and my brother. My fears were allayed somewhat, though, as Mum seemed to cope very well with being single again. Coming from a large and very close family certainly helped Mum get over the breakdown of her marriage. I was confident that she was going to be okay, and she held it all together with aplomb, keeping all three of us above the parapet of a life of struggle and hardship. I don't want to give the impression that I came from an impoverished and broken background, because I didn't. I came from a home of love and support, and there was always a meal on the table at the end of every day. We didn't have much money, but I never went without. What more can you ask for?

When I was 18 years old, I decided to reinvent myself. It's revelation time. And this one, dear reader, is a biggie. I was not born Ellis James Stewart. My birth certificate name is Stuart Carter. My biological father was a chap called Thomas Geoffrey Carter. I have always thought that name made him sound very presidential, like one of the historical founding fathers of the United States. But, alas, he was not. Sadly, he was an alcoholic who succumbed to the debilitating effects of the illness which he lived his life under. When I was born, Mum gave him the simple task of registering the birth at the registry office. My first name should have been Stewart, spelt exactly that way. The Scottish way, on account of the fact that this was my mum's maiden name and my grandfather's family surname. However, my father, slightly inebriated, told them my name was to be Stuart. He returned home with a birth certificate made out in the wrong name and a puppy from a rescue shelter. You had but one job.

I subsequently spent the first six years of my life as the wrong Stewart. Not a great start to life. Thank you, President Carter, aka my real father. My mum loved him, though. She must have, because she married him and then had me. There must have been love from the outset, but when his drinking became too much, that was when Mum packed everything up and we left.

In 1979 my mum had remarried, and I gained a stepdad. He wanted me to take his name, which my mum agreed to, so my name was officially changed by deed poll to Stuart Goddard, my new stepdad's surname. For those of you with a passing interest in '80s pop phenomena, you will have picked up on the fact that this was also the real name of Adam Ant, the charismatic Prince Charming lead singer of Adam and the Ants. It is probably no coincidence that, when I was a small boy growing up, Adam and his band of singing ants became the first band I recall listening to. I remember getting all the records bought for me as Christmas gifts. 'Prince Charming' became the anthem of my youth.

I had this new name for the next 12 years of my life.

It carried me through all my schooling and two years at college. When I turned 13, my mum divorced my stepdad. For the next five years, I bore the name of a man I no longer saw, and who was no longer a feature in my life. Male role models had sadly been lacking from my young life so far. Thank God for Adam Ant and now Andy Bell, the lead singer of the '80s synthesiser-pop duo Erasure. I saw Erasure live twice in my teens, once at Whitley Bay Ice Rink and then again at the Milton Keynes Bowl in 1990. I was such a hardcore rocker back in the day.

Just after I turned 18 and became a man, I decided to act. I no longer wished to keep the family surname of a man who was no longer a part of my life. But this presented a huge problem. Did I become Carter again, as I legally was on my birth certificate? No, I did not fancy that either. I didn't want to be a Carter. I did not even know who this person was anymore. I didn't know a single person from his family. Nope, I decided. My mind was made up. I would adopt my mum's maiden name and family surname of Stewart. Yes, there was one slight problem with this, which you have probably realised. My first name was Stuart. I had my issues growing up, but I did not want to add to them by naming myself, Stuart Stewart. Can you imagine? Something had to give. But what? It was a conundrum. After a lot of soul searching and decision-making, I decided what had to give. It was the name, Stuart. It was the wrong name, anyway, given to me by my drunken father on his way to pick up a puppy. At 18 years old I decided I was going to have a new first name. This was exciting. If you could change your name and call yourself whatever you wanted, what would you choose? That was the decision I had to make when I decided to reinvent myself. From the ashes, this Terminator would rise again. And rise I did.

I was born Ellis James Stewart in a local solicitor's office on 20th March 1992, aged 18. Where did the name come from, you may be wondering? I had absolutely no idea. I just really liked the sound of it. Yep, that's right. I didn't choose it based on anything other than the fact that I just really like it. How's that for reinventing oneself?

I will recap for you, as I know this may have been a total mindfuck. For the first six years of my life, I was known as Stuart Carter. For the next 12 years, until I was 18, I was Adam Ant—sorry: Stuart Goddard. For the last 29 years, I have been known legally as Ellis J Stewart. Stewart is the name my wife and children have. This is who I am.

When I turn 60, I might change my first name again for the twilight years of my life. Hmm! Now there's a thought. I like Maverick, which means independent or non-conformist. A Maverick might just set his own rules in life. Maverick Stewart. Watch this space.

***

Sergeant Dillon. A name that sends shudders down my spine, even to this day, 33 years since the last time I had the misfortune of being in his firing line of vocal and unequivocal, systematically targeted abuse.

I was 14, a mere boy, a quiet and shy one too, when I first had the dishonour of meeting and pissing off a sergeant from a local rival marine cadet detachment. I was a member of the Hartlepool unit. Dillon was an instructor in the Stockton-upon-Tees branch just up the road. Luckily, our paths did not cross all that often. But when they did, all hell would break loose, and that hell was usually unleashed by Dillon in my direction. You see, the man did not like me. That is evident whenever I look back upon this period of my adolescence. To be fair, he didn't like many people. But he particularly did not like you if you were from the Hartlepool cadet unit, which I and some of my peers were.

When the annual camp time came around, you could

bet your bottom dollar that Dillon would be there with his cadets, ready to put the fear of God into any small child who innocently gazed his way. I began to fear going away on these camps purely because I knew he would be there. At six feet, six inches tall and with bulging biceps that could have crushed my little skull like a nutcracker to a walnut, he looked every bit as intimidating as he sounded, with a classic military-style handlebar moustache that would not have looked out of place on an SS officer. I was simply shit-scared of the guy. He had even been blown up in Northern Ireland in his time as a regular Royal Marine. Half of his stomach was missing. He was one incredibly tough so-and-so. I think he often forgot that we were just a bunch of kids and not real Marines.

At the time, my surname was still Goddard, and boy, did I know it. Whenever he saw me, it was, 'Goddard, for God's sake, man, what are you doing?' and 'Goddard, get your arse over here. No, not there! I said here. And be pronto about it.' One thing he would say to me quite often was a reference to my rank. At the time I was a cadet lance corporal, which meant I had one stripe, which I wore on my arm. It was a basic supervisory role among the other cadets, but it gave me a level of seniority over the new starters. If I did something which meant I had messed up, in his eyes at least, he would look me up and down, shake his head in disapproval and then tell me to put my stripe on Velcro, meaning so he could rip my lance corporal rank away and demote me. This was a regular occurrence and his most popular threat.

I wasn't the only one scared of him, either. He had an intimidating effect on a lot of the cadets, including my friend Mark, who, as I was at the time, was also a lance corporal. One incident springs to mind, when we had been away at sea cadet summer camp. We were there that week in the kitchen and dining area, helping to feed and clean up after 200 sea cadets, morning, noon, and night. We were also doing a basic cooking and catering certificate as part of our week-long stay at the camp. Mark and I had been assigned breakfast duty all week, which meant we helped to cook the bacon, eggs and toast and then to serve it up to all of the cadets and officers queuing at the serving hatch. Whenever Dillon would approach with his tray in hand, he had this uncanny ability to make us both instantly fall to pieces.

I was dishing out the sausages one morning, and Mark was serving the eggs. When Dillon reached us, he rolled his head from side to side and drew back his eyes, with a look that instantly let us both know of his disapproval at our very presence.

'Sausages, Sergeant?' I feebly uttered, all the while noticing Mark's hand beginning to shake, the same hand that was holding the spatula for serving up the fried eggs.

'Yes, I will have three please, Goddard,' he gruffly replied.

Now, to this day I don't know what possessed me to say back to him what I did. Even as the words were coming out of my mouth, I knew this was not going to end well.

'You can't have three,' I said. 'You're allowed two maximum.'

Mark stared at me, hand still shaking, his eyes widened. If eyes could talk, Mark's had just said to me, 'What the fuck have you just done?'

There is a scene in the 1981 horror movie, *An American Werewolf in London*, where two friends walk into a pub in the middle of the Yorkshire Moors, The Slaughtered Lamb. As soon as they walk in, the music cuts dead and everyone looks up from their pints, staring horrified at the two young friends for having the audacity to walk into their pub. In an army camp somewhere in Northumberland in the summer

41

of 1987, we had just replicated that scene perfectly, as almost the entire cafeteria stopped what they were doing and gaped open-mouthed at Mark and I, two friends about to be ripped to shreds. But not by a werewolf, although Dillon was scarier than any on-screen monster I had seen as a child growing up.

In a way, I was correct. I was only doing what I had been told by the chef. 'No one gets more than two sausages; we have to make them go round,' he had informed us all at the start of the week. But this rule did not apply to staff. No one told me that, and I had just picked the worst member of staff possible on which to try and enact that rule.

Dillon bore down on me; he leaned down and brought his face to within an inch of mine. My lips started to tremble. Inside my head I was thinking, 'I want my mum.' He began to speak.

'Goddard, put three sausages on my fucking plate, you little shit, or else I'll shove the one you won't give me so far up where the sun doesn't shine that it's not even worth thinking about. Is that clear?'

'Yes, Sergeant,' I replied, tipping all three onto his plate.

'Keep that stripe on Velcro,' he uttered as he moved across to Mark.

On Dillon's tray, there was a cup of tea, a bowl of Weetabix cereal, some toast and the plate with the three sausages on it. Mark asked Dillon if he wanted a fried egg. When he nodded that he did, Mark, with a spatula in an ever-worsening shaky hand, tipped the fried egg clean on top of the bowl of Weetabix. Splat! Milk cascaded over the side of the bowl and onto Dillon's plate of toast. 'Oh, shit,' I recall immediately thinking. Here we go again. But that's not what I said. Oh no, I didn't say anything. I laughed instead. The scariest and meanest person to ever walk this earth had just had a fried egg plopped on top of his bowl of cereal, and I laughed. Surely I was done for.

'Do you think that's funny, Goddard?' he asked in a tone which increased in aggressiveness.

'No, Sergeant,' I shot back.

But the damage was done. He went on to add how he'd been about to make Mark run around the circumference of the entire camp repeatedly, all morning, but instead, I had just taken his place.

Yes, I secretly thought. I didn't mind running. It got me out of the kitchen cleaning duties, and I still had a head on my shoulders. Mark joined in too, to show solidarity.

Dillon became the tormentor of my youth, and I hated the times when we got to collide. Another collision occurred not long after Egg-and-Sausagegate. This time the venue was the beautiful English Lake District. My unit had been camping in the Borrowdale valley, where we had been carrying out practice field exercises. We had been learning escape and evasion techniques, discussing as a large group where an enemy could be hiding, given our current location. Dillon had created a rough map on the ground using whatever we had lying around: a boot brush to depict that forest over there, a few pieces of crumpled brown paper to reflect the hills in the distance, a bootlace for the stream. You know the kind of thing. He asked where the enemy was likely to be. I assumed this was a trick question.

'Here, Sergeant,' I said, meaning exactly where we were standing.

No, not hiding in the forest or wading through the stream, but just here, exactly where we were. Mark shook his head, because he knew what was coming. Everyone else sniggered. By now I was a corporal, which meant I had two stripes on my arm. Dillon was disgusted when I had one; he would flip out if he discovered I now had two. Which he did. I knew it was coming.

'Fucking Goddard,' he began. 'Put those stripes on Velcro, because they are definitely coming off.'

And there it was.

I will never forget the day that Mark finally lost the plot with him. How Mark came away unscathed from the encounter is a mystery to me, even to this day, some 32 years later. Once again, we had spent a torrid time in Dillon's company at a cadet camp. We had taken his shit and his beat-downs and put-downs all week long. It felt like he genuinely had it in for the Hartlepool cadets, which Mark and I were part of. We had to fall in on the parade ground one day for a kit inspection. We were told to assemble with all our kit packed in our backpacks ready for two days wild camping. My backpack was a khaki green, as was everyone else's. Everyone's, that is, except for Mark's. His was the brightest royal blue, the type you would see in a Millets outdoor high-street store. Dillon homed in on him. Mark had made a major mistake that morning. He had left the lid of the backpack open. Dillon flipped it over Mark's head so that it obscured his eyes and began to disperse the contents of his pack all over the parade ground, flinging stuff everywhere. One of Mark's trainers almost decapitated me, missing me by millimetres. I then helped Mark pack it all away again after Dillon had gone.

I can't help but think that if this had gone on today it would have been reported as abuse. But back then, in the '80s, no one said a word. It was normal behaviour.

The evening Mark finally flipped came after a long day of activities outside in the pouring rain. We were tired and irritable as we got ready for bed in our bunked dorm accommodation block. It was five minutes till lights out, and we still had kit strewn around everywhere. We had to sort out our kit, put away all the wet stuff, brush our teeth and then crawl into our pits, all before the lights went out. If we were still up when that happened, there would be trouble ahead. And guess who was doing the rounds that night, making sure all the cadets had hit the sack at lights out? Yep. Dillon. It was time to face the music and dance. For Mark, at least. I completely wussed out.

He strolled into our dorm when we were still faffing about with our wet kit.

'I don't mean to be a pain, gentlemen,' he said, 'but you have exactly two minutes to get into your beds before I beat the shit out of you.'

I flew under the covers, still fully clothed, soaking wet and caked in mud. Assuming Mark had done the same, I was horrified to see that he had not. Dillon flicked the switch. It went dark.

'Mark, Mark, get into bed', I quietly whispered, imploring him to save his own life.

'Fuck him,' Mark replied, not even attempting to silence his voice. 'I've had enough of his shit.'

By now I could tell that Mark was a man on the edge, or at least a 14-year-old boy on the edge. It was an edge that both he and I had been pushed towards all week, and now teetering over the abyss, Mark decided to push back. I was sure this was once again not going to end well.

'Get into your pit, Bradley,' Dillon shouted in the darkness.

'I will in a fucking minute,' Mark shouted back, with anger in his voice.

I was convinced I was about to say goodbye to my friend for good. Any second now, I would see Mark lifted two feet off the ground, with Dillon's fist planted square on Mark's chin. Mark would hit the wall at the far end of the room and then drop to the floor in a heap, sliding down the wall as he went.

Dillon then did something that defied all logic. It proved that maybe he was human after all, and not this evil dictator

45

we had feared he was.

'Okay,' he responded. 'But be quick.'

He turned his back and then left. What the fuck had just happened? I looked at Mark through the darkness without saying a word. He got into bed without saying a word back. I slept soundly that night for the first time all week. The beast had been slain, thanks to my friend Mark.

To this day I will never know why Dillon decided that night not to launch Mark into the middle of next week. Maybe he was all bark and no bite. Maybe he realised we were just children and that it wouldn't look good beating up a 14-year-old. Maybe he had no comeback when challenged. The whole thing happened in mid-December. Maybe it was just a Christmas Miracle. I will never know, and I guess some things are just best left in the past. Life moves in mysterious ways.

I never did put my stripes on Velcro, and I never lost them, either. I even gained another one, becoming a cadet sergeant before I finally left. Dillon would have been furious.

When I look back on memories such as this from my life, it makes me realise that although at the time it was traumatic and stressful, it also became character-building. It left no lasting damage on my psyche. Not to my knowledge, anyway. Mark should know, as he became a Consultant Counselling Psychologist in his later life. We often look back on these years and have a chuckle together. This is usually over a drink. Isn't that strange? Events that scared me senseless as a small boy are now memories which elicit feelings of nostalgia. Reminiscing about this time never fails to put a smile on my face.

CHAPTER TWO
MY LIFE AS A POWERMAN

'Voyage upon life's sea, to yourself be true, and
whatever your lot may be, paddle your own canoe.'
Sarah Bolton

In the mid-90s I fell in love with a sport which was frenetic,
unconventional and just simply glorious. Originating in
China, this sport would give me a sense of pride and
purpose for the first time in my life. I discovered what true
teamwork and camaraderie meant. I also became a British
champion.

My first introduction to dragon boat racing occurred
one weekend, shortly before my time as a Royal Marine
cadet had ended. I took part in a charity boat race located
in Hartlepool docks. Each dragon boat consisted of 14-20
paddlers sat next to one another in a longboat. A dragon
boat is essentially that, a boat designed to look like a
ferocious dragon, with a large neck and head at the bow of
the boat and a tail in the stern. A drummer sits at the front,
beating out the rhythm, while a steerer stands at the back,
making sure the boat stays in a straight line, much the same
way as the oar is used as a rudder on a gondola in Venetian
canals. In-between the drummer and the helm steering, the
paddlers sit in twos, propelling the boat to the finish line as
quickly as possible. It is quite a spectacle, and the races are
absorbing and exciting to watch, let alone to take part in.

The sport made its debut in the UK in an episode of the BBC's *Blue Peter,* way back in 1986, when a boat was raced from London to Nottingham, paddled by soldiers for the Sport Aid charity via the UK canal system.

Sitting in a dragon boat that weekend at the cadets as a geeky and gangly 14-year-old, I had no idea I had just discovered a new sport which, over several years, would go on to captivate me.

As we would quickly learn, it wasn't as easy as it seemed. It was all about timing. The key to moving the boat forward as quickly and efficiently as possible was by striking your blade into the water at precisely the same time as the person sitting in front of you and the person sitting behind you. This timing was critical to the success of the boat slicing through the water. Get it wrong and you soon knew about it, when the paddler behind would clatter his paddle into your hands. As we moved across the water, reminiscent of the way a caterpillar moves across the land, I became aware of a team next to us who appeared to be good. Actually, they were really good and easily crossed the finish line, with our team some distance behind.

Every other team that weekend, us included, was truly awful. At the end of the racing, I struck up a conversation with one of the paddlers from the winning team. He informed me that his team consisted of employees from a nuclear power plant up the road. They had been racing dragon boats for a few years on the national racing circuit and had become one of the top racing teams in the UK. This came about after they entered a team to take part a few years earlier in the European Dragon Boat Racing Championships in Belgium. What had started as a bit of a jolly, and a weekend away with the lads on the drink, ended up becoming something of a different proposition altogether when the team from the power plant only went and won the thing, becoming European champions! I had to laugh when the guy I was conversing with told me how some of the European teams, in their skin-tight spandex suits, with protein shakes in hand, were left bewildered and gobsmacked that twenty fairly unfit power station engineers from North East England, with beer tins in hand, had raced the event drunk all weekend yet somehow still prevailed, victoriously. When a chap from Hartlepool says they are going to do something, generally they do it.

Figuring that, as a non-power station employee, I wouldn't be able to join the team, I forgot about the whole thing for a year or two and decided instead to devote my time to other things. But my time in a dragon boat would eventually come, and with it so would that British Championship medal. As the team was predominantly funded by Nuclear Electric, the parent company of the power station, it stood to reason that you needed to work at the station or at least know someone who did to stand a chance of breaking into the team. As luck would have it, though, my friend Mark got speaking to a guy in the gym where he trained, who happened to mention that he was a member of the team and that we were both welcome to try it out ourselves. Mark, like me, had also been in that dragon boat race at the cadets all those years ago, and was as keen as I was to see if we could make the team.

Although it would initially take me a few years to prove my worth and force my way into the team, I still turned out three to four times a week and gave it my all with the training. This included two to three sessions a week out on the water and one session in a gym doing circuits and general fitness. Mark was also hammering away at it, but his fitness was far more telling than mine, and he quickly established himself as a regular paddler with the team. I had to work a bit harder to stake my claim.

My friend Mark Bradley and I were not only in the cadets together, but we were also at the same school. I first met Mark on our very first day at secondary school. I was standing around in the yard along with all the other new starters, nervously waiting for the bell to ring so we could enter the school.

Mark wandered into the yard, and someone shouted in that cruel way that only cruel kids can, 'Ha, look at Bradley's flares!'

Indeed, he had the widest bell-bottom trousers on of any kid that day, but he took the insult in his stride, and quick as a flash quipped back, 'Piss off.'

I liked him instantly.

Mark was also one of those two friends who went into the Royal Marines. However, due to a slight short-sightedness with his vision, he was told that he could do the training and duly pass out, but he would then have to become a chef or a desk clerk. For someone who had visions of becoming a PTI (Physical Training Instructor), this left a bitter taste, and he promptly withdrew and ended his short-lived career as a Marine. As someone who also did disastrously badly at school, he came out of the Marines and quickly set about correcting his academic shortcomings.

Even today, I still call Mark my friend. After 36 years of friendship, we are still very close. We both have our family homes on the same road in the same town. Mark did indeed slay the demons of his school education and progressed through to the highest echelons of academia by earning a doctorate and becoming a Consultant Counselling Psychologist. Not bad for someone who left school with as appalling an academic record as I did.

***

In my early 20s, I felt very sheltered and very naïve. I didn't have much life experience, and I wasn't well travelled. I had never even been on a plane. All that would change, though, when I finally broke into the dragon boat crew, just before my 21st birthday. I was now officially a member of the Hartlepool Powermen Dragon Boat Team.

We competed far and wide, both domestically in the UK and overseas, when the opportunity arose. The team was predominantly made up of employees from Nuclear Electric, who at the time had the contract to run the operations of the nuclear power station, a few miles up the coast from Hartlepool. With the nuclear industry receiving negative press, the company saw any positive story as good PR and used the success of the boat team as marketing gold. If the team kept winning, then Nuclear Electric was willing and able to keep pumping money into supporting the crew. Consequently, in a sport that was expensive to compete in, we became the richest team on the circuit. Whenever we would go away to races, we would always rock up in a nice big fancy team coach, like a Premier League football team. We would stay over in the nicest hotels and wine and dine on pretty much whatever we fancied. We were hyper-disciplined when we needed to be, though, and there were many occasions when we trained and lived like Olympic athletes, especially in the run-up to major races, such as the National Finals.

The team of which I was now a member was invited to compete in an international festival in Vancouver, Canada, in the summer of 1994. I was possibly more excited about the prospect of my first time on a plane than I was the actual event. The seven-hour flight to Canada was my very first experience not only of flying but of cabin-crew hospitality too, and not one to be rude, I took full advantage of this, as did the rest of the team. It is fair to assume that, as a team of reasonably grounded young men, we could party as hard as they come, but equally, when the moment called for it, we would be the consummate professional sports team, where not a single drop of alcohol would cross our lips for days, even weeks.

On the evening we landed in Vancouver and collected our luggage, we were informed in the airport that we would need a police escort to our hotel in the heart of downtown Vancouver, as a disturbance was currently in full swing. Unbeknown to us, the Vancouver Canucks, the city's ice-hockey team, had just been beaten in the Stanley Cup Finals by the New York Rangers. This had led to large scuffles, and at times violent confrontations, between the police and up to 2,000 fans outside the stadium. As the game ended, it was reported that up to 50,000 to 70,000 ice-hockey fans had converged upon the downtown Vancouver area. This soon became a riot, as shops were looted, and cars and buses set on fire. Riot police used tear gas to disperse the crowds.

We made our way to our hotel, passing the heart of the rioting and fighting, through a dense fog of tear gas. One of the rioters saw us in our team tracksuits and started walking towards me.

'Hey man, where are you guys from?' he asked.

I rather nervously informed him that we were from the UK and that we were here for the Dragon Boat Festival.

'Cool, man. My girlfriend is from England,' he replied, before mentioning that he hoped to live in the UK once he had finished his college degree in humanities. 'Good luck and enjoy Canada. You'll love it here,' he said as he shook my hand.

He then proceeded to light a rag hanging out of a bottle of some spirit or other and hurled it towards an oncoming police car, where it bounced off the windshield and rolled into the gutter.

There are certain things and experiences in my life that you just cannot make up. This was one of those times. As we were nearing the entrance to our hotel, a sports shop next door was being looted and ransacked right before my very eyes. A glass cabinet of Oakley sunglasses came crashing out onto the sidewalk, spilling its contents right across my path. I was horrified. We just did not see this kind of thing where I grew up in England.

The following morning, after the riot had died down, I strode out into the street, looking for somewhere to have breakfast. I put on my brand-new Oakley sunglasses, while shaking my head in disbelief at the night before. Shocking, I thought to myself.

***

Racing in Canada was a real eye-opener for us. Up until that point, we had felt we were a decent team, which we were, to be honest. If we lost a race, we usually lost by the slimmest of margins and would generally exact our revenge the next time we raced. However, in Canada, in front of thousands of spectators and a TV audience in its millions, we were brought crashing down to earth as we were comprehensively out-paddled by a team, the majority of which paddled for the Canadian national squad. By comparison, we were just a ragtag bunch of engineers and welders from a nuclear power plant. It was like Bayern Munich playing a part-time Sunday league football team. The outcome would be as you'd expect. Complete annihilation. We had been humiliated and schooled in a sport we thought we were good at. The Canadian team, which was one of the best in the world, had finished the race, were out of their boat and sunbathing by the time we crossed the line, such was their margin of victory.

Realising just how far off an elite level we were, when we returned to the UK, Nuclear Electric agreed to cover all the costs of bringing over the coach of the Canadian squad for a week-long intensive training camp. This proved decisive for the team. Later that year, at the National Championships, we were runners up.

The following year, we wiped the floor with every team we raced, which finally culminated in winning the National Championships. The races took place at The National Water sports Centre, at Holme Pierrepont in Nottingham, where it had been held for several years previously. The team had been close to winning on several occasions but were constantly playing catch up to a canoe club from Kingston-Upon-Thames. In the autumn of 1995, though, it all came together, and several years of hard work and dedication were rewarded when we crossed the finish line one nanosecond ahead of the Kingston crew. We went through the entire season unbeaten.

When I look back on my time in the team, it's easy to say we were good because of this or because of that, but I think I can put the majority of the success down to one thing: our coach, Dave Price. Dave worked at the power station as an engineer, and he had even got his wife Jean to join the team as our drummer. But in Dave, we had a natural-born leader. He oozed leadership ability, and he ran the team with a style of leadership I had not seen before or since. His pre-race team talks were legendary and would not have looked out of place in the changing room of any elite-level sports team. 'You must be elated at how much you are dicking everyone this weekend,' he once said after an event in London where we had beaten everyone we raced. To combine humour with motivation is a rare talent indeed. But Dave could do it effortlessly. He needed to, as we were a raucous bunch, and he had to get our attention somehow. Humour, particularly toilet humour, would always do the trick. It is testament to how good a leader he was, though, that when the time came to be serious, we would all give him our undivided attention. Sometimes you would have been able to hear a pin drop during one of his motivational talks. In Dave, I discovered an individual who would go on to inspire me in so many ways. I was a relatively quiet and shy member in a team which had some larger-than-life characters. I was always happy to keep quiet and take a back seat, largely so I wouldn't become the butt of a joke or two.

***

Life in the team had gone too smoothly for too long. With most things in my life, and as if to restore some equilibrium, another misadventure is often just around the corner. And that proved to be the case with dragon boat racing. In my Everest book, I fleetingly mentioned about the time I had almost died in a freezing-cold lake in the English Lake District, in the dead of winter. I dismissively said perhaps I would save that story for another book. Well, guess what?

They say that when you're about to die, your life flashes before you. That didn't happen on the day I almost died on Everest, but it did on the day I clung to the underside of an upside-down dragon boat on Derwent Water in northern England. It was a day when the entire dragon boat team almost paid a premature visit to the pearly gates.

We were competing in a new winter series of races in lakes and rivers around England, while the main racing season had finished with the culmination of the national finals in Nottingham. Normally, a race distance during the normal season would consist of short sprints of 250, 500 and 1,000 metres. The race distance that day on Derwent Water was 10,000 metres, to one end of the lake and back. We arrived that day as cocky as ever that we would win. We went home with our frozen peckers between our legs, well and truly reminded by Mother Nature who was boss. The race should never have been allowed to start. Derwent Water, which is usually a tranquil body of water with a mild current, looked like something akin to the ocean waters around Cape Horn. The water looked mean and menacing. The waves crashed all around in every direction.

It was a miserable, grey, wet, cold and windy day. A normal day for the English Lakes, you could say. We arrived, got our boat in the water and began warming up. Kitted out in just our usual race kit of skin-tight, body-revealing Lycra shorts and vest, we were no match for the weather that day. There was certainly no place to hide your modesty in this kit. For such a tough bunch of blokes and girls, it was also quite camp. And it had a pink stripe, too. Several crews began the race. We were determined to be the first crew past the post. Only minutes into the race, other crews began capsizing after being swamped by the tsunamis coursing down the lake. Our goal suddenly changed from winning the race to being the only crew to finish it. Someone shouted from the back of the boat, 'They started this race, we'll finish it.'

At the time, we had a status of being the best racing crew in the whole of the UK. We had a fierce reputation. Train hard, race harder, party even harder. We had even become minor celebrities, after appearing on the ITV Saturday night game show You Bet, hosted by Matthew Kelly. On that occasion, we had successfully completed our challenge by pulling a double-decker bus down a runway, attached by a pulley to our boat in a lake next to it. The BBC wildlife presenter Michaela Strachan was our celebrity backer. At the time, she was married to a chap from Hartlepool. She famously said, when asked by Matthew if she thought we could do it, 'When a man from Hartlepool says he is going to do it, then he does it.' I fancied the pants off her. She was also the presenter of a late-night dance show called *The Hitman and Her*, which was always on TV when you stumbled home from the nightclub at 3 in the morning with a doner kebab slopped all down your front.

As we paddled down the lake that day, I remembered her words: 'When a man from Hartlepool says he is going to do it, then he does it.' I almost stood up at one stage and screamed in a Mel-Gibson-as-William-Wallace-Braveheart-style war cry, 'Do it for Michaela!' but then I realised this was a silly thing to do. So, I stopped myself before I stood up and capsized the boat. The balance was critical in a dragon boat. Even just someone shifting their bum in their seat could affect the stability of the boat. As the race progressed, things went from bad to worst. Somehow, we had managed to remain upright and still afloat. We had made it to the far side of the lake, where we became obscured back to the starting area by a small island. By now, we were the only remaining crew in the race. All the other teams had capsized within minutes of starting. Most of the rescue boats were by now busy extracting cold paddlers from the lake, who had been in the water for a few minutes.

If we could keep paddling forwards, we had no problem. But we were heading towards a huge problem. The same way a passenger plane can overshoot a runway on take-off and landing, we were running out of a lake with which to paddle in. The end of the lake was fast approaching. We would need to turn and head the other way to complete the return journey. For the first part of the race, we had been paddling with the waves. They had been propelling us along and helped to keep us buoyant. We had as much chance of turning a 40ft-long narrowboat with twenty paddlers a full 180 degrees in these conditions as we did flying it to the moon. But we had to.

Our helm, Joe, gave the order to turn. 'Brace the boat, get ready.' We began the turn.

Miraculously, we somehow managed to get the boat pointing in the opposite direction. We were now heading towards the finish line in the right direction. But to reach the finish, we would need to use all our strength to paddle against the biggest waves in an inland lake I had ever seen. Not that I am an expert in inland lake patterns. Almost immediately, we began taking in water. We were fucked! Like the scene from the George Clooney and Mark Wahlberg movie *The Perfect Storm,* about a commercial fishing vessel that was lost at sea in a storm in 1991, we began climbing almost vertically up a wave.

'Come on!' I shouted, in one last act of defiance.

But then, like the Andrea Gail, the ill-fated ship from that movie, we began sliding backwards. This is not good, I thought. Seconds later, we were underwater. The boat was gone.

When I came up to the surface, I immediately began hyperventilating. The cold penetrated every inch of my rapidly freezing body. I couldn't get my breath. This, in turn, was forcing me to panic. Crew members all around were scrambling to grab onto anything. Someone grabbed onto my back, which forced me back under the water. Luckily, a split second later, our boat re-emerged, half-submerged and upside down, but floating, nonetheless. We all scrambled for it, clinging on to the side of the boat, which was now a good few feet under the water. The problem was, to hold onto the boat and stop ourselves drifting away into the lake, we had to endure the water continually washing over our heads.

We had by now been in the water for almost five minutes. Already, I had lost sensation in my body. In water this cold, the human body has minutes to survive before the bodily organs start to shut down. Because the extremities start to freeze, blood rushes out from the core to try to warm up the fingers and toes. But this leaves the core vulnerable. Hypothermia is a certainty.

We would later learn that some of the crew members from the other teams who had capsized almost at the start would suffer from mild hypothermia. They were in the water for five minutes at the most. By now we had been in the water for ten minutes, and there was still no sign of any rescue boats coming to our aid.

I was in my twenties and in great shape, but I was struggling. Some of those in the boat were much older than I was. At one stage, I suggested trying to make a break for it and swim to the lakeside, which looked tantalisingly close. This was instantly dismissed by some of the more senior members of the crew, who recognised I would have no chance in currents and waves this strong. I was glad it was. I didn't fancy my chances, but something had to happen, and soon, or else we were done for.

When some of our crew started to let go of the boat and close their eyes, it all became a game of life or death. Throughout the whole ordeal, one of the things I recall being frustrated about was being able to see the lakeside and land. I could see cars on the road that skirted the lake and lights on in buildings and farmhouses. But we might as well have been in the middle of Cape Horn. 10 minutes became 15, which became 20. Dave, our coach, started to worry, not so much for himself, I thought, but for the fact that he also had his wife Jean in the boat, as well as his daughter Jodi. He had also allowed his young son Adam in the boat for the first time. Thankfully, Jodi and Adam both wore wet suits, which offered them some protection from the rapidly declining conditions. I could still see the worry in his face when I glanced at him. My friend Mark Bradley was counting out loud. At the time I thought this was odd. I thought maybe he was delirious with the cold. He later told me he needed

something to focus on to keep his mind away from the penetrating cold. With some of our crew now being unconscious and held out of the water by some of the stronger members of the team, we had minutes left. We had been in the water a full 25 minutes.

Finally, we heard the dull drone of a boat's motor speeding towards us from the far side of the lake. Sweet Jesus, we were going to be saved. The rescue boats had not been aware of our predicament because they could not see us. They had estimated when they thought we should be back at the start area. When that time had come and gone, they realised something was up and came looking for us. A flotilla of boats emerged at the scene and began scooping us out of the water, one by one. None of us could help, as we had no control over our motor skills. Numb and floppy bodies were dragged out of the water and into the back of the boats. Our rescuers then got to work on trying to warm us up. I had a foil blanket wrapped around me, and several people began to rub my body to try and get some circulation going. All the while they were asking us our names, and ages, and where we were from. When we made it back to the start area, ambulances had already been put on standby to whisk us away to the infirmary in nearby Keswick.

Everyone who had gone into the water that day suffered from the effects of hypothermia. Some fared better than others, while for others it was a very traumatic experience. For a good while after the event, some of the members of the team could not bring themselves to talk about the events without becoming emotional.

I was informed afterwards that I had the three best-looking female rescuers attending to me in the boat racing to shore. I was completely oblivious to this point. That probably explains why they were able to rub my groin with no reaction at all. We all eventually recovered from our ordeal with nothing more than bruised egos and perhaps hatred for lakes, in winter, in horrendous conditions.

***

Sometimes in the darkness, we must find the light. And I found that light in the form of Jean's drumstick. Jean, Dave's wife was the team's drummer. To beat the drum, she needed a drumstick. Some mischievous but skilled carpenter had made Jean's look like a large penis. I spent the journey to shore staring at an eight-inch-long wooden penis. Yep, I've said it before and I'll say it again, life moves in mysterious ways indeed.

Dave Price would ultimately go on to coach the Great Britain men's national dragon boat team. When he eventually took early retirement from his job at the power station, he moved into human performance coaching in the nuclear industry. He travelled the world and made a fortune. I still see him to this day, as his daughter Jodi married my friend Mark. We tend to meet up at Christmas time in the local pub, where we reminisce about the amazing times we all had as a Hartlepool Powerman. We rarely talk about Derwent Water, though. That is a memory best kept locked away.

The last time I shared a beer in our local pub with Dave and Mark was Christmas Day, 2018. I had to leave unceremoniously without even putting the beer to my mouth. Tamara called me in state of panic, to inform me that our kitchen was on fire.

'Crap, I have to go, guys,' I said as I stood up and flew out the pub doors.

'What's going on?' I heard Dave ask with concern in his voice.

'Oh, nothing much,' I responded. 'Just my house on fire!'

That was a Christmas day to remember. The firemen

managed to save most of our house, with only the downstairs affected. The actual fire was caused by yours truly. I had lit a scented three-wick candle and placed it on a windowsill in the kitchen. This was to provide a pleasant vanilla and cinnamon odour to disguise the smell of the turkey roasting away. Unfortunately, I forgot to tell Tamara—who was upstairs in the shower—that I had lit a candle before I left to walk to the pub. My youngest, Isla, wandered into the kitchen as the three wicks merged into one.

'Err, Mummy,' Isla shouted upstairs. 'I think there's something wrong with this candle,' she added in a slightly more concerned voice.

Tamara ran downstairs with one towel around her hair and another around her midriff, just in time to see the wooden blinds on the window go up in flames. Woosh! It happened as quick as a flash. Flames began to lap across the ceiling of the kitchen. It was at this point that Tamara realised any effort at trying to put out the flames was futile. She closed the kitchen door, got the girls and the dog out of the house and rang the fire brigade. She then rang me. I sprinted all the way home. When I arrived, all our neighbours had come outside to see what the commotion was. Tamara stood shivering, still dripping wet from the shower, dressed only in two towels. She did not look amused.

'Merry Christmas,' I said, before throwing my arms around her.

At least they were all out of the house. At the end of the day, a house is just bricks and mortar and stuff. It can be replaced. Human life cannot.

When our neighbours' 4-year-old son asked for a fire engine from Santa that year, I don't think he was bargaining on the real thing turning up outside his house. He was over the moon.

When the fire had been safely extinguished, we were allowed in to assess the damage. Bizarrely, the turkey had carried on cooking away, despite the raging inferno all around. We were entertaining that year and were cooking dinner for Tamara's family. They all turned up an hour later. Sitting eating Christmas dinner in the charred and dripping-wet remains of our dining room is an image that will live long in the memory.

***

Life is full of misadventure and mishap. You can attempt to climb the highest mountain in the world when an earthquake strikes, you can paddle a winter boat race dressed in nothing more than revealing figure-hugging lycra, or you can be a total jackass and light a candle, then leave to go to the pub, inadvertently setting fire to your kitchen on Christmas Day. There is never a dull moment.

CHAPTER THREE
MY WORKING WOES

'Hard work never killed anybody,
but why take a chance?'
Edgar Bergen

I have done it all. And I literally have done it all. As I
stated at the start of this book, I am a Jack of no trades,
therefore definitely master of none. My working life has
been as eclectic and random as it's possible to get. Now,
this is all well and good, from the point of view that I have
experienced a lot of variety. But I would not endorse this
way of life. It's very unsettling; just ask my long-suffering
wife Tamara. I didn't set out for this to be the pattern of my
life. I think, in a way, that maybe it chose me. Or more to
the point, the universe decided I would drift around, trying
different vocations, and never really settling in anything of
note for an extended period. Why? I don't know. In 30 years
of work, this has been the constant question I have tried
desperately to answer.

For 29 of those 30 years, I have searched within myself
to come up with that answer. In the last year, I have now
stopped trying to solve the riddle. I have accepted that
this is who I am. A leopard cannot change its spots. You
cannot fight fire with fire, and no matter how much a snake
sheds its skin, a snake is still a snake. And despite my best
efforts to the contrary, no matter how much I sought a

conventional career path, it didn't and hasn't happened.

Does this mean I am a screw-up at life? Have I failed in my role as a man, as a husband, a father, a son, a lover, a friend, a hunter and a gatherer? Hey, Ellis, welcome to Loserville, where the population is you, you dumbass. I guess this all comes down to perspectives. Right now, my perspective is one of optimism and renewed hope. I am bursting to the brim with faith and belief. I know that sounds like I am about to become all high and mighty and start spouting the Bible, but I am not a very religious person.

However, I do believe in something. I think the universe has our back. Whenever I have prayed in my life, I have never prayed to God, the Lord above. But I do send my prayers out into the universe. When it comes to God, I take the agnostic point of view. I would like to believe, as we all would, that there is a higher being and that we are all being watched over and guided through our journey of life. But I am not so sure without concrete proof. I am not an atheist, though.

Where does my faith come from, then, if not a god? I feel that something or somebody watches out for me. Of that, I am convinced. That same somebody or entity that continually tells me no, but sometimes says yes. No, you don't need to get into debt to buy that brand-new Jeep. No, don't drink that sixth pint of beer, this will only end badly for you. No, you should not skip that five-mile run and eat a Big Mac instead. Running shoes on and get your arse out of the door.

We all hear that voice in our head. The voice of reason, the voice that pulls us back from the brink and saves us from making stupid mistakes. Occasionally, though, even the voice in our head can trip out and tell us that it's okay to stick another £2k on a credit card. What? You want to buy the latest Apple iPad because yours is a few years old now? Do it. You know it makes sense. You are a bit peckish? Order a large greasy doner kebab immediately, with a side serving of chips and wash the lot down with a keg of beer. A 5-star spa break for the weekend, you say. Sure, you need to spend £1000 on a few nights away, rejuvenating. Who cares if you only have £100 to your name right now? Your body needs this, damn it, stop being selfish to your body.

You see, sometimes the voice gets it wrong as well as getting it right. This is the same voice that tells me to walk out of a job after only one day because it 'didn't feel right.' Yes, I've done that. I've also done all the above. Damn you, voice, I thought you had my back.

When it comes to the world of work, I often listen to that voice, but occasionally I let intuition take over. I fly by the seat of my pants and throw caution to the wind to see where it will take me. And I have had quite the adventure—sorry, misadventure—in doing so. In no particular order, some of the jobs I've done over the past three decades include:

***

Paperboy, glass collector, mobile DJ, club DJ, hardware store assistant, campsite activities instructor, campsite barman, record store assistant, outdoor store assistant, outdoor store assistant manager, outdoor clothing sales rep, warehouse worker, snowboard store assistant, visual merchandiser, call centre agent, life skills coach, taxi driver, stationery products delivery driver, Amazon delivery driver, (lasted one day), worked in a gas plant as an energy trader, screen printer, sold T-shirts on eBay, sold T-shirts on Amazon, sold merchandise at running events, public speaker, motivational speaker, inspirational speaker, absolutely wonderful speaker, book author, trek organiser, book author again.

Every single one of these roles I have undertaken has left a mark on me and made me the person I am today. Some I heavily regret doing, some I had nothing but joy doing. Some I am still trying to do. Hey, Ellis, what do you do for a living, again? I am an entrepreneur, remember. Oh yes, you did say. So, you are unemployed? What? How dare you!

Some of the more regrettable roles I've had didn't start that way. The regret ended up being the main takeaway, due to the outcome. Throughout everything I have ever done to bring in the dollar, I have carved my own path and danced to the beat of my own drum. I have been respectful when I've needed to be, disrespectful when it is warranted and resourceful and diligent to the umpteenth degree. If you are being paid to do a job, then do the job. No half-measures. But I draw the line at being courteous to cretins, and I will not kiss the arse of some jumped-up, egotistical little prick just to climb the ladder.

In my working life to date, I have made thousands of people dance to the music I played, I have shown eight-year-olds how to build a raft and then seen the glee in their eyes when they sail that raft. I have told a shop manager to shove his job where the sun doesn't shine and walked away with not a jot of remorse. I have driven a car for 20 hours straight and then watched the most spectacular sunrise. I have inspired, motivated and entertained thousands of people, all through the power of my words of adventure. I have made small children laugh and grown women cry. I have sold snowboards to snowboarders and whiskey to alcoholics. I have taken people to the hospital in the back of my cab and been propositioned with sexual favours when other passengers have had no cash to pay the fare. I have designed clothing that gives people hope and ambition and sold my designs to all corners of the world. I made £4,500 from an email and £1,500 for a 20-minute talk. I have written a bestseller about failure and traded gas through the early hours of the night.

These are all life-defining moments that are the essence of who I am. We could all paint a picture with words which describe our working lives. How many pictures will be as varied as mine? Sometimes you must take a chance and live a little. You do not need to have your whole life worked out by the time you are 21. I am 47, and I still don't know what I want to be when I grow up. I am thinking of becoming either a rock star or an astronaut. I haven't decided yet. I still have plenty of time.

And that, right, there is completely the right attitude to have. Always be ready to learn and ready to take chances when opportunity strikes. Always be willing to improve and willing to discover new things about yourself. There is so much of who I am that I have learned from what I do and from who I meet along the way.

I appreciate that my way of being is not everyone's cup of tea. There is a certain lack of stability and security that tests the most resilient of minds. In 2002, I was down on my luck, one of the many times in my life when I've had the ignominy of being so. I had moved back up north to County Durham a year earlier and spent the whole of the year working in a call centre. It was a gloriously underpaid position, doing work no one wanted to do in an industry no one wanted to work in, all the while being appreciated by no one, not least the customers I would call and harass daily. I was keen to leave as soon as I could. The opportunity to do so came my way when I applied for and was offered a job as a life skills coach for a young person's charity. The job title sounded way more impressive than the job itself, but I was willing and keen to give it a go, plus it got me away from the phones in the call centre. Working with the disaffected and disadvantaged youth of the North East, my job was to provide and teach them basic life skills.: opening a bank account, basic budgeting and planning, maths and English skills, how to be an upstanding member of society, that kind of thing.

These 16-year-olds had been booted out of mainstream education for a whole range of behavioural issues. Expelled from their schools, no college or prospective employer would take them on. They had to go somewhere; we were that somewhere. They would be paid £30 a week to attend for 16 hours a week. They needed to attend the full 16 hours to be paid the money. There was a slight problem, though; none of them wanted to attend, and often they didn't. On the off chance that they did show up occasionally, they would become as disruptive as they possibly could, in the hope that you would send them home. Which normally worked.

I wish I could say I spent a long and happy time working for the organisation, being able to inspire the youth of the day to become better and more rounded future adults. I lasted two weeks, and that felt like a lifetime. I could not get through to them. I had no teaching skills I could fall back on, and I couldn't manage their unruly behaviour very well at all. A 16-year-old girl in the group taught me more swear words in one day than I knew existed; the same 16-year-old girl who would later headbutt a boy because he fancied her.

They were an unmanageable and wayward bunch, who came from a background of broken homes, abuse, neglect and foster care. They were the forgotten generation that no one wanted to deal with. Except they had to be dealt with. If all of society turned its back on these young people, they would become feral, lawless and most probably homeless.

When not teaching life skills in a classroom, I would drive them to places such as bowling alleys, indoor football courts, cinemas and swimming pools. The list of where we could take them was getting smaller by the day. Everywhere I took them we would then be subsequently banned from. At the bowling alley, one of the boys from the group thought it would be funny to throw himself down the lane rather than the bowling ball. He smashed into the pins with his shoulder, sending them flying. It wasn't even our lane. It was the lane next to ours, occupied by a family. I was so embarrassed. I offered a thousand apologies before we were ejected from the premises. This pattern continued everywhere we went.

The best thing to do was to keep them in the classroom at the centre, away from members of the public and public facilities. One day, the charity had arranged for a so-called 'expert in problematic teenagers' to come in for an afternoon and carry out a workshop, which he guaranteed would motivate them to think about their actions. I spoke to the chap beforehand in the kitchen, where I made us both a drink.

'So, you think you can get through to them?' I said as I handed him a steaming hot cup of coffee.

'Yes, I know I can,' he rather confidently answered back. 'It's what I do'.

He packed up and left less than an hour later, covered from head to foot in the cup of coffee I'd made for him. One of the little darlings had flung his backpack at him after being told to be quiet.

As the expert strode past me, I heard him mouth under his breath, 'The little fuckers! Unbelievable.'

If an expert couldn't reach them, I had zero chance. I'd been getting paid to take abuse in a call centre less than a month ago. In this new role, I felt totally and woefully underprepared. I was no match for what these 16-year-olds could dish out. I was hopelessly out of my comfort zone. As luck would have it, I didn't need to wait too long before an end to my misery came along. I was fired at the same time as I resigned, sensing I was not cut out for the role. The 'fired' part came about for assaulting a parent and destroying company property.

One of the lads, the alpha male of the group, had brought a bag of cannabis into the building one day. I found him in the toilets making up a joint, ready to pass around among a few of the other alphas of the group. When I challenged the group, I immediately received a mouthful of obscenities. I managed to grapple the drugs away from the ringleader and perpetrator of the crime. I informed him that it was confiscated because it was illegal to bring drugs into the centre. I tried to take the moral high ground and give the group a stern talking-to about the harm that taking drugs would do to them.

'It's a slippery slope, lads,' I offered up to bolster my stance. 'You'll start on cannabis, and then before long, it will be cocaine and heroin. No good will come from it.'

I could see my remonstrations were falling on young, ignorant and deaf ears, so I stopped trying.

I took the bag of cannabis and locked it away in my desk drawer, all the while facing a barrage of protests and insults from the lad I had taken it from. I didn't have a plan for how exactly I was going to deal with the situation. I think, ultimately, I would have informed my line manager at the end of the day and hopefully got an answer as to the correct course of action. But the end of the day never came. At the first opportunity he got, the young lad ran out of the centre and then ran the short distance to his home to tell his dad I had stolen the drugs from him. Later that afternoon, the lad and his dad stormed into the centre, looking mighty angry.

'That's him over there, Dad,' the lad shouted, pointing directly at me.

The dad stormed over to me. 'I hear you have something

that belongs to us. I want it back, right now.'

I stood up from my chair and walked round to the other side of my desk, so I was now only a few feet away from the guy. His face as red as beetroot, I could see veins throbbing in his neck and forehead. He certainly didn't look like the type of guy you wanted to anger or piss off. By confiscating his son's bag of narcotics, I had clearly done both.

'You can't have it back,' I said. 'It's illegal, and he shouldn't have brought it into the building.'

I braced myself, wondering how dad was about to react. I knew he wasn't going to say, 'Ah okay, fair enough. Come on, little Johnny, let's go home. I did ask.' Bear in mind this was a father who didn't have a problem with his seventeen-year-old son having drugs in his possession and using them. A split second later, the dad grabbed a tight hold of me round my T-shirt collar, forming fists which lifted me onto my toes.

'Give me back the fucking gear now before I knock you out.'

Yep, that was pretty much what I'd been expecting. I adjusted my feet to stabilise my balance and stop myself from tumbling backwards. I managed to get both my arms out in front, and in one big effort with both hands, I pushed the dad in the centre of his chest to try and get him to release his chokehold from around my neck. I didn't think it was that forceful a push. But it was. He flew around six feet backwards, stumbling and flailing about as he went, completely losing his balance. He crashed into the wall on the far side of my office and continued going. The office was a small, fabricated construction within a much larger building. The walls and ceiling to the office were very basic and quite flimsy, as I was about to find out. When Dad hit the wall with his back, that entire side of the office began to fall backwards. It happened in slow motion. It reminded me of the way a tree falls after being chopped down with an axe. I should have shouted 'TIMBER!' as a warning to people on the other side. CRASH. The wall hit the floor of the main building, sending a plume of dust into the air. At that exact moment, the wall to the left of where I was standing began to topple backwards too. Once that wall hit the floor, it was inevitable that the ceiling was going to give way, bringing with it the fluorescent lighting tubes.

The whole collapse seemed to take ages but must have been no more than a couple of seconds. Once this domino effect had stopped its path of destruction, I was left standing in front of my desk, where my office used to be. Two of the walls that had just seconds before been standing now lay flat on the floor. The ceiling had snapped clean in two. Broken glass from the shattered lighting tubes was scattered everywhere.

Dad had by now stood up and was about to launch himself at me for Round 2, but the rest of the centre staff had been alerted to the office collapse and had raced over. It would have been hard not to be alerted; it must have sounded like a bomb going off.

The boy's dad was restrained until he calmed himself down, all the while reiterating over and over how he wanted the bag of cannabis back. This drew attention to the fact that I may have been in the wrong for taking the drugs. I was told to report to the head office immediately to discuss the chain of events that had just occurred.

Dad shouted at me as I left, 'If I ever see you again, I'm going to smash your fucking head in.' He definitely had a way with words.

In the office, I had a meeting with the manager of the charity for the entire North-East region. I explained what had happened about taking the drugs and how the office collapsing was an act of self-defence. An incredulous laugh resulted.

'You call that self-defence? I would hate to see what would have happened had you attacked him,' he said.

After almost accepting my version of events and agreeing that there was no malice intended from my actions, he went on to say how we could not be seen to have staff members attacking students' parents. It wouldn't do the reputation of the charity any good, he further added. I couldn't believe that they were siding with the boy and his moronic, irresponsible lout of a father.

'I'm afraid this is as far as your journey with us goes. I am going to have to let you——.'

Before the words had finished leaving his lips, I interrupted. 'Don't worry. I quit.'

And that was that. I had lasted all of two weeks and three days in my new career as a life skills coach. Looking back, I felt it was such a shame that things had ended the way they did. I had a lot of life skills that I could have taught and imparted to those unruly youngsters. The only problem was, they did not want to listen. You can lead a horse to water, but a pencil must be lead.

Without a doubt, the worst job of my many varied and multiple multi-skilled career choices began in 2002. I had just turned 29, and I still had no clue what I wanted to be and do in my life, or how to achieve it. I had recently left the call centre and been fired from/resigned the life skills tutor role, and I was looking for a fresh challenge. I had started dating the previous summer, and I was still somehow in that relationship a year later. Tamara put up with a hell of a lot when we first met. She still does, if I'm honest. With one eye still firmly on cloud-cuckoo-land, hoping I would be off to climb Mount Everest soon, I half-heartedly began a new job search.

A friend of mine had recently started driving for a new start-up taxi firm in my hometown, and one day, over a coffee, had told me how they were still taking drivers on. Excellent I thought. I'm going to become a taxi driver. If it's good enough for De Niro, it's good enough for me. Yeah, okay. Just one problem with that way of thinking; Hollywood is always so different from real life, as I would discover.

Be that as it may, I still enthusiastically signed up for a licence with the local council, and I had to wait a few weeks before the licence came through. I then sat a basic test of my local geographic knowledge. This was a little bit like the test that cab drivers have to sit if they wish to work as a cabbie in London, except it was much easier, and also nothing like the 'The Knowledge' taxi test. With the test passed and licence secured, it was time to begin my taxi driving misadventure.

I knew that being a cabbie was only going to be a short-term fix. I was still planning on going off to Everest one day, and I had now also started looking at returning to school, more specifically going to university. But I still threw myself into the job with excitement and hope. Besides, I was broke and needed the money.

It only took two weeks for that excitement and hope to be crushed. How I would go on to do the job for over a year and a half is, quite frankly, a mystery.

A taxi driver will either work days or nights. Days are generally more relaxed and stress-free, whereas nights are more hectic and livelier. Day-shift driving would, however, mean fewer earnings and more traffic on the roads, plus it took twice as long to get to where you were going. Nights, on the other hand, offered more earning potential and quieter roads. It was simply a case of choosing your poison. I chose nights—more specifically, weekend nights.

On a typical Friday or Saturday night, I could expect to earn between £100 to £150 a night in takings, that is the total of passenger fares. The taxi company whose car I was driving around in would rather generously allow me to keep 30 percent in commissions. Basic maths meant £100 on my worksheet, £30 in my back pocket. You would add to this by acquiring tips that passengers would either give you or, nine times out of ten, not. Sometimes you could double your take-home pay. If you were very lucky, you could go home at the end of one of your shifts with around £80 in your back pocket. This doesn't sound too bad, but when you then factor in that this amount is earned across a 12-hour driving shift, it starts to look—well, a bit shit, which it was.

It didn't take me too long to cotton on to the fact that, as a new driver, and one who chose to only drive weekend nights too, I was well down the pecking order when it came to being looked after. Loyal drivers, those who had worked for the firm for many years, and full-time drivers were the ones who made the most money in fares. I also quickly discovered that out-of-town jobs were the most lucrative. I could earn the same amount of money taking a passenger to Newcastle Airport—a journey of around two hours there and back—as I could spending five hours driving around the town. Because of that, I craved the out-of-town work, more so than picking up Betty, a 90-year-old serial gambler, who would spend every night of the week dipping her weekly pension into the slot machines and dabbing away at the prospect of a full house at the bingo hall.

One of the reasons why I chose to drive nights was to avoid the Asda supermarket pickups. I absolutely hated these types of jobs. I would pull up in the taxi bay outside the supermarket and then get out of the car and shout out the name of the passenger I was there to collect.

'Jones,' I would shout, then wait a moment for no one to approach. 'JONES,' I would scream again, before finally seeing my passenger approach the car with three trolleys' worth of groceries, fit to bursting.

'Eh, sorry there, love, I didn't hear you.'

I would pack all the groceries into the boot of the car, drive to the other side of town, unload the shopping and carry it up two flights of stairs, before placing the bags in the customer's hallway. Technically, I wasn't allowed into a customer's home, which I would occasionally need to remind them of. There were some passengers who, I am sure, would have loved nothing more than for me to go into their home, put away all the shopping, make them a cup of tea and put slippers on their feet before leaving.

For all my efforts on one of these supermarket jobs, I would earn the princely sum of 66p, no matter how long it took or how many miles I drove. If the passenger lived within the town, they qualified for a daytime-shopper special for the bargain price of £2.20. Daytime ended at 6.00pm, as did all the special fares. As soon as I realised this, I changed my shift start time from 5pm to 6pm. Goodbye shopper specials, hello night-time rowdiness.

For the next 16 months, between the hours of 6pm and 6am on a weekend night driving that taxi, I would experience more real-life than in the first 29 years of my life put together. One of the many jobs I undertook included being used for a drug run. I was given a small brown bag and an address to take it to. I then had to drive back to the original address and hand over the money from the Francis Begbie lookalike from *Trainspotting* who had swapped me it for the brown parcel.

That same week, a few days later, I was used as a getaway car driver. Three guys, clearly in a panic, jumped into my cab one night when I was sitting at a junction.

'Drive, drive!' one of them barked at me. 'Go, go!' said another, and all three clearly looked keen to leave the area as soon as possible. I did what all drivers would have done in my position. I floored it. I never did find out what they had done. To be fair, they paid the fare and tipped rather generously.

I had people pee in the back of the car, throw up in the back of the car and even poop in the back of the car. I was propositioned with offers of sexual gratification in exchange for the fare, but I declined. I had people run away without paying, and I even had someone pull a box-cutter knife and demand all my takings. I called his bluff, and he ran off. The worst of humanity was thriving in my days as a taxi driver, and I generally gave it a lift.

A girl once got in the back of the cab who had just been beaten to within an inch of her life. She was as black and blue as the colour of the cab I was driving. When I offered to take her to the hospital, she point-blank refused. I asked her who had done this to her, which again was met with a stony resistance. She wouldn't talk. I called the police after I had dropped her off and gave them her address and the address where I had picked her up from.

I knocked a girl over who, arguing with her boyfriend, ran out of her house and straight into the path of the taxi. She bounced off the bonnet, landing in a heap on the road. When I went to see if she was okay, I was told to 'Fuck off' and that she was fine. So off I fucked, albeit with a now-damaged taxi.

But the undisputed, no-questions-asked, mother of all my taxi pickups occurred one evening after I had been sent on a job to pick up a female passenger by the name of Pat from a pub. This was to be my last fare that evening. It had been a particularly quiet shift, so I had decided to finish early, promising myself that this was to be my last job. It was midnight when I arrived at the pick-up, a rough-looking public house that had seen much better days. It was in an area of the town which was generally regarded as being no-go once it got dark. You just didn't know who you would meet outdoors once the sun went down.

My fare was escorted out of the venue, held up by two members of the pub's bar staff. Pat had both of her arms draped over each of their shoulders. She was a big lady who had seen much better days. She also looked as though she had consumed her body weight in alcohol, judging from how out of it she appeared. We all helped to get Pat into the back of the car. I was given a ten-pound note and her address. It was a short five-minute journey, with the sound of loud snoring coming from the back seat to keep me company. Outside Pat's house, I tried to summon her from her deep sleep and get her out of the car and into her home. But I was not having much luck. Eventually, a neighbour came out of a nearby house after hearing my engine running. 'Come on, let's get you in, Pat, you big daft bat,' he said as he helped to get her out of the car and standing up straight.

No sooner had we got her standing up straight than she fell backwards. It was sickening to watch. Like the office walls in my previous job, it was like watching a tree topple. 'TIMBER!' Only this time it was a human being falling. Pat hit the ground with a sickening thud. Her head cracked back on the tarmac of the road. Immediately I saw a pool of blood begin to flow from out of her matted dark hair. 'Oh, shit.' I had experienced many interesting fares in my time on the taxis, but I had never had a passenger die on me. I was determined that this wasn't going to be the first time.

All I had in the boot of the taxi was a tartan dog blanket, which I placed on the back seat. The neighbour said he would call for an ambulance. I figured it would be quicker to drive to the local A&E department, which was literally and luckily just around the corner from where I was. I asked the neighbour to help me get her back in the car. Using all our strength, we were able to do so. I supported her head with a car-cleaning sponge after checking she was still breathing. With Pat back in the taxi and bleeding heavily from a nasty gash on the back of her head, I Starsky & Hutched it as fast as I could to the hospital.

I screeched up outside the doors of A&E and ran to the front desk.

'I have a female passenger with a serious head wound,' I said to the girl behind the desk.

She looked at me in horror. Everyone began to stare at me in horror.

'Are you sure it's not you?' she said, looking me up and down.

I was covered in blood. It was all over my jeans and my T-shirt. I looked as though I had been put up against a wall and a firing squad had let rip on me.

A paramedic followed me out to the car and then went back into the hospital for a wheelchair. After he had examined Pat's head wound in the car, I once more helped to get her out of the car and into the wheelchair. At the exact moment we got her in the chair, she started coming round. She tried to stand, but the paramedic forced her back down.

'Stay where you are, we need to see to that head of yours,' he said.

Pat was becoming more lucid by now. She clocked me and once more tried to stand. 'Hey, handsome,' she said, 'give us a kiss.' She puckered up her lips and started making kissing sounds through them, before she began laughing hysterically. 'Hey, he's a bit of alright, him, isn't he?' she said to a female nurse who was now also attending to her head.

Pat was covered in blood; it was all over her face, her hands and her blouse. She kept pushing hair back from her

81

eyes, and every time she did, she would smudge the blood that was on her face. She looked like a character from *The Evil Dead*.

As she was finally wheeled away into the hospital with a tartan dog blanket wrapped around her shoulders, she inexplicably began singing. 'Hey hey, baby. Uuh, aah. I want to know oh oh oh oh if you'll be my girl.'

I arrived home at 3.00am, after spending an hour scrubbing blood out of the back seat of the taxi. After showering, I fell asleep to the sounds of that song repeating in my head.

***

The Christmas shortly before I stopped working as a taxi driver, I worked on Boxing Day. The taxi company would pay 50 percent commission over the Christmas shifts, and the fare was double time, so there was money to be made. I worked my socks off all day long. Starting at 11.00am, I drove all the way through till 2.00am the following morning. I was ready to log off, happy with the 15 hours I had just driven and the money I had made as a result, when I decided to accept one more job. Big mistake. As a part-time driver, I had never been offered many of the lucrative out-of-town jobs, instead, I would pick up all the drunks and waifs and strays around the town and take them from door to door. It wasn't very lucrative, but it was steady and reliable.

I have no idea why the dispatcher that night decided to give me my first real out-of-town job, at two in the morning, after I had already been on shift for 15 hours straight without so much as a coffee break. I accepted the job offer that had flashed up on my screen, not knowing where I would be going till I accepted it. It was Manchester Airport and back; more specifically, taking a family to the airport to catch their flight for a winter break. This meant I would be in the taxi for at least another five hours. It was a one-way, two-hour drive at least. From Hartlepool, you would drive down to Leeds then across the M62 motorway through the Pennines.

I picked up my radio and I dialled in to speak to the dispatcher.

'Er, about this job you have just offered me,' I said. 'You do realise I have been working since 11a.m. yesterday?'

A loud sigh came over the radio. 'I do, yes. Do you want it or not?' the dispatcher said with impatience in his voice.

Even though I was dog tired, I did want it. The fare was £140, and I would earn half of that. I started to reason with myself. So that is £70 for around 4 hours' driving if I am quick, so that equates to £17.50 an hour. I quickly worked this out in a few seconds flat, even in my tired state.

'Fine, I'll do it,' I answered.

The journey to the airport was not that bad, as I had the family I had picked up to chat with. The journey back was a real struggle. I pulled into motorway services, doped myself up on coffee and Red Bull and drove home most of the way in a blizzard with the window open, allowing the freezing winter air and snowflakes to drift into the car to keep my mind sharp and active. It did the trick; I pulled back into Hartlepool at exactly 7.00am, a full 20 hours after I had begun my shift the previous morning. The sun was just starting to rise over the sea, so I parked up and watched the most spectacular winter sunrise I had ever seen. I need to find a real job, I recalled thinking as I drifted off to sleep.

I endured some memorable nights as a taxi driver, none of them good ones. When I finally started a university course several months later, I decided it was time to quit to concentrate on my studies. At least I wasn't fired this time. I can never be accused of not working hard—when I work in the first place, that is.

Throughout my working life, I have made some good impressions on people, and I have made some not so good. I have possibly been fired more times than I have quit. It is true what they say: most people work just hard enough not to get fired and get paid just enough money not to quit. It is perhaps no coincidence that the jobs I have been unceremoniously let go from have been the jobs I didn't care for. Getting fired has also been a blessing in disguise, ultimately leading to bigger and better opportunities. Even Steve Jobs went on record as saying being fired from Apple was one of the best things that could ever have happened to him. He said it freed him to begin one of the most creative periods of his life. He was re-employed a few years later and helped to launch the iMac and the iPhone. The rest is history.

While I haven't gone on to create anything as ground-breaking and revolutionary as the iPhone after I have been fired from some of my roles, I do feel that I have become a better person for it. I was fired from my first ever job after school for telling the store manager of the DIY hardware store I was working at to go and fuck himself after he would continually ask me to run around after him. The final straw came when he asked me for the third time to get him some toilet roll so he could blow his nose. The first two times I complied, the third time he felt my wrath.

I was almost fired from Our Price records in Milton Keynes, a temporary Christmas position I had started as my first job since relocating from the North East to be with my then-new girlfriend. I was working upstairs in the '60s, '70s and '80s CD department. One of the store supervisors had taken a dislike to me, which I detected when she said to me on one shift, 'I don't like you.' Say it like it is, I recall thinking. Don't beat around the bush.

This made for an uncomfortable working relationship,

until I finally had a run-in with her. She had chastised me in front of a customer for placing a Simply Red CD into a case for the Beatles' *Sergeant Pepper's* album. Luckily, the customer noticed and returned it to the store immediately. It was an innocent mistake.

I jokingly said to the customer, 'What's the matter? Do you not like ginger hair?

I laughed, and so did the customer. My supervisor didn't.

'So, you think that's funny, do you?' she said as she stared me down.

She then called me an arsehole in front of the customer. I was a bit speechless. I did not know what to say. Looking back, I don't think that saying what I said helped the situation any.

'If I'm an arsehole, then you are a complete bitch,' I said.

The customer hurriedly left, looking rather embarrassed.

I was hauled in to see the manager, who gave me an official warning and told me it was my last chance.

'My last chance? What about her?' I offered up in my defence. 'She called me an arsehole—in front of a customer, too.'

The supervisor was also given a warning. Yes, karma is sweet.

The most unfair dismissal of my working life came shortly before I had moved down to Milton Keynes. I had taken a job working the whole of the summer in a caravan and camping park in the Lake District. By day I would run the children's activity club, and by night I would work in the club's bar. Entertaining kids in the daytime and serving the parents alcohol at night. It was a great job, and I thoroughly enjoyed it.

It was time at the bar one night, and a chap approached, wanting to buy a bottle of wine. I told him that I couldn't serve him anymore, as it was now after-hours. But he would

85

not take no for an answer. He kept pleading with me to sell him the wine. In the end, to shut him up I gave him the wine and took the money. The tills had now been closed for the evening, so I had nowhere to put the money. I placed it into the bar staff's communal tipping jar, of which I would take an equal share. The bar manager had secretly watched the whole transaction unfold. The following morning, he had removed me from the rota for the rest of that week. When I challenged him on it, he told me I was a thief, and that he would not have thieves working in his bar. My pleas for leniency fell on deaf ears.

Later that day, I quit the activities job, packed up all my stuff and caught the last train from Penrith to Buckinghamshire. The indignity of it all was too much to bear.

***

I haven't been fired from every job I've ever done. There have been certain jobs which I have thrived at and loved every single moment of. One such job was Total Warrior.

Total Warrior is a large, mass participation, obstacle-running race which takes place in northern England. For five years, I supplied all the event merchandise, which I sold from a marquee in the event village during the weekend of one of their events. The event was held in three locations: Yorkshire, Cumbria and Edinburgh, and I loved every single one of them. I was not directly employed by Total Warrior, but my printing company, of which I was the director, had been given the contract to supply all the event merchandise. This meant creating and designing the products, working out what I thought I would sell at an event and then hopefully selling everything at the event to the participants and spectators. I did a pretty good job at this. A weekend at a Total Warrior event would see, on average, upwards of 6-8,000 participants and 20,000 spectators. With this many people visiting the event village, I realised I was going to need a team around me to help me staff the marquee.

I started working with Total Warrior in 2014. Not being sure how many staff I would need and how much to pay them, I did what everyone in my position would have done; I asked my family to help me out for the weekend instead. I had just returned from my first attempt on Everest, so everything was a tad chaotic and disorganised, but we came through the weekend in fine style. I was also allowed to run the race too if I wished, as was anyone else who worked on the merchandise stand. I couldn't see my 66-year-old mum plus her sisters wanting to run the race, but my 21-year-old cousin Nathan was game, so we ended up running the race together while my mum and aunts manned the stand.

I thought that my family helping that first event would be a one-off, to help me get started and find my feet. But when the next event rolled around less than two months later, they were as keen as mustard to return and help again, as they had loved being involved that much. Far be it for me to rock the boat. This worked out in my favour and turned out to be a shrewd move on my behalf. My mum and aunts did not want paying for giving their time for free for each event. All they asked was that I covered their expenses during the events, which for five ladies in their sixties amounted to nothing more than several cups of tea. I also offered to cover any petrol costs, accommodation and evening meals.

For five years, it was a total blast. We all had so much fun. It never felt like work, as the vibe of the weekend was so friendly and positive. Whenever a Total Warrior weekend was coming around, I could sense the excitement building with my mum and her sisters. I made them staff uniforms when I realised that they were in it for the long haul. This mainly consisted of a T-shirt which had Total Warrior Merchandise Implementation Team printed across the back.

I'll give those ladies their due, they certainly knew how to sell. At every event, my cousin and I would take part in the race, while the ladies would sell, sell and sell some more. We would get close to selling out of everything we brought to every event. What we didn't sell, we could roll over and take to the next event. It was very rewarding, seeing a design I had produced on my computer back home being worn on the backs of thousands of participants and their supporters, not just at the events but all around the UK.

One of the enduring memories of Total Warrior was watching my mum (who had never taken part in a running race in her entire life) at our last event in 2018. After five years and over sixteen events, she had become a fountain of knowledge on breathable and wearable technical sportswear. By the end of my time with Total Warrior, she and her sisters could have peddled snow to an Eskimo.

'Now, this a wickable, 100-percent breathable, polyester top,' she said to two young male runners who had been browsing in the marquee. 'It's guaranteed to make you feel comfortable out on the course.' She always had a habit of bringing me into the conversation. 'If you don't believe me, ask my son Ellis. He has used these tops on Mount Everest, don't you know.' Then she would add, 'Ellis, tell these fine young men all about how comfortable this top is.'

It was a joy to watch her at work, and I was very proud of her. I was proud of all my family for helping me out when I ran Total Warrior's merchandise. For the last two years, my Aunt Pam's 70-year-old husband Dave got involved. He had a particular talent for selling hooded sweatshirts, so that became his department. He became my Hoodie Houdini. Like the famous escape artist: now you see me, now you don't. With Dave, it was now you see this hoodie, now you don't, the speed at which he could sell them.

Everyone was sad when I decided to stop working with Total Warrior. I felt it had run its course, excuse the pun. The event was changing too. They had gone down from three events to one, reinventing themselves as the obstacle course Great North Run, just once a year. I knew it was time to depart, and in 2018 we bowed out after five great working years with the guys and girls of Total Warrior. And there was not a single firing in sight.

***

Getting the contract for Total Warrior had come about because of the printing company which I'd started out of university, several years earlier. Myself and my friend Steve began dabbling in T-shirt designs in 2006, the year we both would graduate from our courses. I would graduate with a first in Business, thanks to Steve helping me out with one of the accounting modules I found tricky. Steve earned a 2:1 for his degree and got less in the exam he helped me out in than I did. I continually rib him about this, but Steve would get the last laugh, going on to earn a fortune in the city as an energy trader. I remained, hopelessly, a lost cause.

The company that we started that year was christened Toffee Monkey, on account of Steve being an Everton football fan, nickname the Toffees, and myself being from Hartlepool, nickname the Monkey Hangers. It was the perfect amalgamation of names, and we had burnt the midnight candles coming up with it.

We bought ourselves a basic printer and heat press from eBay and a CD of designs. In the Christmas of 2006, we sold hundreds of T-shirts on eBay, all copyright breaches and all ripped off from other designs we had seen. The first T-shirt we sold had an image of the actor David Hasselhoff across the chest, with the words Don't Hassle the Hoff. It was genius, and we sold hundreds.

It was only when an official letter came through to us

from the legal representatives of The Rolling Stones that we realised we might be doing something wrong.

'I told you we shouldn't have sold those Mick Jagger T-shirts,' I said to Steve.

We paid back the near £1,000 fine for breaching the Stones' intellectual property rights and realised we would have to change if we were to make a success of this business. Steve, realising that if he could not sell T-shirts with pretty much whatever he wanted festooned across the front, decided to bail out and stick with his real job. I, on the other hand, decided to rebrand and continue. And so, Planet Adventure was born. Now staying on the right side of the law, I began to create my own unique and often humorous designs. As sales increased, I started to investigate splashing out on better equipment. For a good few years, the business boomed. I went from being a sole trader to a limited company in a very quick timescale.

Christmas was always the busiest time of year, and I would do almost half my year's turnover in just two months. One-year sales were so good that I was processing around 100 sales a day. On December 12th of that year, I suspended my online operations to concentrate on dealing with the backlog of orders, which I could not keep up with. I took on extra staff around Christmas to help, but it was still tough going. All told, that Christmas was the busiest and most profitable period of Planet Adventure's existence. In a year in which I turned over £60,000, almost a quarter of that turnover had been generated from just November and December.

Most of the sales came in from two platforms: eBay and Amazon. The website I had created brought in few sales. Unfortunately, to get the sales and to get your products seen, you needed to be on one of, or ideally both, these marketplaces. And this was the kicker. I gave away a lot of the profits in listing and selling fees. I was mainly selling T-shirts—and lots of them—at £10 each. By the time I had deducted shipping costs, eBay or Amazon fees and the card processing fee, I was lucky if I was left with £3 in profit. The year the business became VAT-registered, I would then need to put an additional 20 percent aside to give to the taxman. I quickly realised the business was not viable. It was hard labour producing the T-shirts, too. I began to hate all the monkey-see, monkey-do, hands-on nature of the business, and it was beginning to wear me down.

I decided to change tack, and instead of selling direct to the consumer, I went for the business market instead. I also diversified the niche into sporting apparel, aimed squarely at the sporting market. This change of direction brought Total Warrior on board and several other smaller events whose interest was piqued by the way I worked with Total Warrior.

During the two years when I went off to attempt to climb Everest, I had added a whole range of designs and clothing themed around the mountain and, as I have alluded to previously, the sales of these helped me to raise a large portion of the expedition costs.

It was one of these Everest designs that led to the best business transaction I concluded in my time running the business. I was on holiday one summer with Tamara and the girls, and I had left the business in the capable hands of my young cousin Nathan. I had told him not to worry and that there wouldn't be much to do, as it traditionally went quiet through the summer months.

He contacted me one day to tell me I needed to check my email. A technology company based in California by the name of Xilinx had taken a liking to one of my designs and wanted to place an immediate order for 300 T-shirts, to be sent to their offices in the US. This was a headache, but it was workable. I told Nathan not to panic and that we could do this. I then contacted some of my aunts who had worked with me on Total Warrior. Nathan knew how to print the T-shirts and my aunts would help him fold and pack the order. Once he had done this, I told him to let me know and I would arrange the international shipping. That is what we did; everyone came together, and I coordinated things while walking around Disney World on my summer holiday. It was a great order and at last some nice recognition for one of my designs.

When I arrived home, I investigated the company background and could see why they wanted the T-shirt. It was worn at a sales conference on the west coast of the US for the launch of a new software product called Everest. They'd ordered the T-shirt with no interest in the mountain at all. For them, it just synced in nicely with the launch of their new product. I didn't mind; it was still my first large international order.

Later that same year, around November time and completely out of the blue, the Executive Assistant to the office of the corporate vice president of Xilinx got back in touch with me and sent me an email. The first question I thought of was why Americans always have great sounding jobs. If this company were based in the UK, the email would have been from the Secretary to the Assistant Manager. I recognised the name as being the same person I had spoken with back in August for the order of the 300 shirts, which Nathan and my aunts had taken care of.

'Hi Ellis,

Your Everest T-shirt was the talk of the town at our last regional sales meet up and product launch in San Jose in September 2016. I would now like to place an additional order for the same T-shirt but in quantities of 1,500. We would like these sent to several of our corporate locations around the world, and they would need to be at each location by December 2nd. I trust this would be okay for you.

Best Wishes, Sarah Lopez'

I checked the date. It was already November 17th. There was no way I would be able to print 1,500 shirts and then guarantee they would arrive at the locations she had specified in a little over two weeks. This had the potential to become the largest single order that my business would ever process and fulfil. They had not even quibbled on the price of £20 per shirt, which was what they had paid for the 300 a few months previously.

If I could somehow pull this off, the order was worth £30,000. I spent a restless day and a sleepless night looking into whether it was possible to fulfil the order. No matter how I dissected it and examined its viability, I came up against brick wall after brick wall. There was just no way I could do it. I was saddened, because I desperately wanted the order. A piece of artwork I had knocked together almost a year ago in Photoshop, which had taken me fifteen minutes at best, was now potentially about to bring £30,000 into my business. I bet some full-time artists spend their entire careers creating designs to sell and never get anywhere near that amount for a piece of their work. This was just stone-cold luck on my behalf, and I was not even an artist, I was a self-taught graphic designer, a basic one at that. At last, was my luck changing? Or should I say, would it be changing if I could work out how to print 1,500 shirts and send them, guaranteed to arrive in two weeks, to seven countries dotted across the planet?

I couldn't take the chance. It wasn't going to happen. But then, in a pure lightbulb moment, an idea came to me. What if I were to license the design for their exclusive use. It didn't matter to them what the garment was that the design was printed on. The design was the key ingredient to the whole mix. If I licensed the design to them, they could then utilise local printers and have the garments printed up in the locations where they needed the T-shirts. It was a brilliant idea of mine—no, scrap that, it was genius. If Sarah and her VP would agree to pay me a licence fee, I would send them an agreement, agree on a price for each shirt that they planned on printing—in this case, 1,500—and then send them the artwork. Voila!

I realised that I wouldn't be taking the full £30,000 that I could have, but I would still be making a sizeable profit, and in the words of one of my favourite North-East bands, Dire Straits, it was money for nothing.

The next day, I put the feelers out to Sarah, with my suggestions. She came back to me straight away and was delighted with my idea. It was going to save them a fortune, and ultimately, name a company which doesn't want to save money. I needed to now come up with an amount and then draft it all up in a posh-looking Word document.

As I was not going to be doing any work whatsoever, other than pushing a 'send' button in an email, I didn't wish to exploit the situation too much. It would have been criminal of me to say £10 per design. That would have been £15,000 in my back pocket for essentially emailing a piece of clip art. I could not have lived with myself. I decided upon £3 per shirt that they would print. £4,500 felt much less criminal and was a figure I was much more comfortable with.

I gave Sarah the numbers, which she instantly agreed to. Damn, that was far too easy. Perhaps I should have said £10 after all. All that was left to do was draft the agreement and send the artwork across. I had never written or even seen a licensing agreement before, so I knew I would have to do some research. As I saw things, I had two options. I could consult the services of a lawyer who specialised in such matters, to help me put together a slick-looking legal document to protect my piece of clip art. Or I could download a template off the Internet and plagiarise it. Guess which option I went for? And it didn't involve a legal fee.

I sent across the document to Sarah's email the very next day.

'Please read this EULA (That's an End User License Agreement, for all you novices) carefully, as it sets out the basis upon which Planet Adventure will license the use of its Everest One Dream design for use by the XILINX corporation.'

It was a three-page wordy document with the above as the introduction and was littered with a profusion of posh and legal-sounding vocabulary and jargon. It mentioned intellectual property rights, the licensor, patents, trade secrets, unfair competition rights and termination contracts. I couldn't have done a better job if I'd tried.

I sent it to Sarah to sign, which she duly did. A few days later I had £4,500 sitting in my bank account, and Sarah and XILINX had the best design I had ever created because of the most profitable email I had ever sent.

A month later, Sarah got back in touch to share several photos of the events around the world. In every one were smiling employees of XILINX, rocking my Everest design. At long last, I was finally experiencing an up in my life. Things had gone my way, and Lady Luck herself had shined on me.

***

My working life has been as eclectic as they come, and I wouldn't wish to change a single moment, experience or firing from any of my résumé bullet points. Benjamin Franklin once said, 'It is the working man who is the happy man. It is the idle man who is miserable.'

The money I earned from the US tech company sure beat driving that taxi around and taking poor old Pat to hospital. I would have had to work 100 shifts in the taxi to earn what I had just done with one email. It certainly made me feel like bursting out into that song.

'Hey hey, baby. Uuh, aah. I want to know oh oh oh oh if you'll be my girl.'

CHAPTER FOUR
MY ROAD LESS TRAVELLED

'Normality is a paved road.
It is comfortable to walk,
but no flowers grow on it.'
Vincent Van Gogh

I was a very late starter in life. I have always done things
well past when I should have done them. Did I pass
my A-Levels aged 18? Nope, not me. I was 23 when I
finally did. Did I get a degree at 21? Nope again. I got my
degree results on my 33rd birthday. And it's the same with
travelling. I didn't start to travel and holiday in my life until I
was well into my twenties. I have since felt very blessed and
lucky that I have, though.

One of my regrets is that I never travelled for an
extended period when I was a lot younger. I wish I had
taken off and explored the world for a year after college
and before I went to university, as a lot of young people
do these days. But then the gap for me between leaving
college and eventually going on to university was 11 years.
And in that time, life got in the way. Yes, I know, I am
making excuses. If I had wanted it, then I could have
made it happen. At the time it was not even on my radar.
I didn't fly until I turned 21. Travel for me as an 18-year-
old consisted of a trip to McDonald's in my clapped-out
banger of a car, 10 miles up the motorway and back.

That was a real adventure.

I didn't have many holidays, growing up. The last holiday I remember going on as a child was a week's camping in the south of France when I was around 12 years old, with my mum, stepdad and brother. This involved a 24-hour coach journey down to the Mediterranean. I remember gazing out the windows in awe and wonderment when the coach drove through Paris, late at night. Seeing the Eiffel Tower was a real treat.

It would be almost 30 years till the next time I went on holiday—the type where you get to relax on a beach, eating delicious food and drinking fine wine in the sun. This was with Tamara when we first started dating. It was the summer of 2002.

I had been to Argentina, Nepal and Tibet a year earlier, but those trips were for mountaineering expeditions. They were not relaxing holidays in the slightest. But that was what I thrived on. Adventure and hardship were my middle names. Lying on a sun lounger doing nothing was not.

Tamara and I went to the Greek Island of Crete the summer after we had met. This was my first ever beach holiday. Two whole weeks of doing absolutely nothing. I remember Tamara packing two suitcases, one for her clothes and things, the other full of books. Why are you taking all those books? This is a bit odd, I thought at the time. It was only after we'd been there a few days that I began to realise: Oh, so we literally just lie around the pool all day doing nothing? I get it now. I was a complete holiday novice. I was as wet behind the ears as it was possible to be.

On that first holiday, I ended up getting completely wasted on my birthday. We had a table booked in a restaurant for 7.00pm. I was very excited; it was the finest restaurant on the island, with breath-taking views of the sea. We stopped at a cocktail bar beforehand. After perusing the drinks menu, I opted for a Zombie, which sounded exquisite. It was that nice that I decided to have two more. When we stood up to leave, I realised I was in trouble. We made it to the restaurant. Just. When the main course was placed in front of me, I was as deathly pale as the fish on my plate. Tamara thought the whole thing was hilarious and laughed hysterically at my pitiful state. Luckily, a power cut hit the island, and the restaurant was plunged into darkness. We both used the opportunity to sneak out before we had even had a mouthful of food. Tamara had to hold me up all the way back to the apartment. I was fast asleep by 8.00pm, and even that was after I had vomited twice on the floor of the bathroom. Happy 29th birthday to me.

After a week of doing nothing, I could take no more. I wasn't used to doing nothing. 'That's it,' I said. 'There must be something to do on this bloody island.'

A day later I dragged Tamara out on a 16km walk through a national park called the Samaria Gorge. I was in my element, Tamara not so much. In the 44-degrees heat, she had a really difficult time of it. We ran out of water halfway through the gorge and had also forgotten to pack sunscreen. When we finally emerged out the other end of the gorge at the Libyan Sea, Tamara could hardly walk and was severely dehydrated.

'Are you okay?' I reluctantly said, sensing how pissed-off she looked.

'Don't you talk to me,' she snapped back.

I didn't blame her, to be honest. All the girl wanted to do was go on a relaxing and romantic break in the sun for a few weeks. It wasn't her fault her idiotic boyfriend had coaxed her to go for a day trekking in the mountains in the blistering heat. We did get to swim in the Libyan Sea with a cold bottle of beer afterwards, so she quickly forgave me.

***

I have always been okay with extremes of temperatures, whether that be on the side of a mountain in Argentina in minus 20 degrees Celsius or the middle of a desert in Africa in 48 degrees, as recently proved to be the case on a family holiday to Egypt.

We had booked to go to the Red Sea resort of Hurghada for two weeks of sun, scuba diving and fun fun fun. We booked to stay at a hotel which looked like Disney's Cinderella castle on steroids. As the holiday progressed, the girls, including Tamara and my mum, who had come along with us for the holiday, were having a fabulous time of it. There were plenty of pools and water slides to occupy the girls and keep them entertained. After I had read the first two Game of Thrones books from cover to cover, I was starting to become irritable.

'There must be something else to do,' I said to my mum and Tamara when I could take no more. Tamara must have thought to herself, Please God, no. Why can't he just be content with relaxing? She looked at me as if to say, 'Don't even go there.'

'Why do we have to do something?' she said. 'Just chill out and be happy.'

In 2017 the United Kingdom government still had Egypt on its beware-of-travelling list, due to recent terrorist attacks in the nearby resort of Sharm-El-Sheik. In fact, Sharm was still closed to UK travellers. We had taken advantage of great price drops to holiday in Egypt, as a lot of people were staying away, fearing a repeat of the attacks. As a result, armed guards were patrolling our resort, and whenever you left the hotel to venture further afield, you needed to have your wits about you.

'That's it,' I said after the sixth straight day around the pool. 'There must be something to do around here.' I went and found the tour guide, who had been walking around the pool all week with a clipboard selling his day packages of fun and adventure. Tamara and Mum both shook their heads in disbelief.

Agreeing to consider booking something, Tamara wanted to travel for five hours in a private taxi 300km to see the Valley of Kings in Luxor, which we were thankfully advised against by the concierge of our resort. As much as I would have quite liked to see the valley, there was no way I was going to sit in a stuffy cramped car for five hours there and then five hours back, just so we could see a few tombs cut out of a rock face. I told Tamara as much. With that ruled out, we looked at other options.

One trip that caught my attention was a full day in the desert, an hour's drive from our resort. It was as action-packed as they come. We would travel in 4x4 jeeps out to the desert, where we would then get to take part in quad biking, before visiting a Bedouin village for lunch and mixing with the locals. This was right up my street. After lunch, we would travel further into the desert, where we would hike up a nearby mountain and then get to drive sand dune buggies. If you think of what a moon landing buggy looks like, then that's exactly what these were, except built for sand rather than lunar surfaces. They looked so much fun. I had an image of flying through the air after launching from a large sand dune. The day would conclude with a late evening dinner and entertainment under the desert night sky and a million bright stars. The whole thing looked brilliant. I was hooked once I saw that it included quad bikes. Everything else was a bonus. After convincing Tamara and my mum that I would be content if they would say yes to us all booking up, they relented and agreed.

The following morning, we had an early breakfast and met outside the resort to be picked up by our transportation. As there were five of us, we had a jeep to ourselves. The journey started quite sedately as we followed a long, straight road out of our resort. After about half an hour the driver suddenly took a sharp left turn and took the jeep off-road, straight into the desert. He then floored it. My mum, Tamara and the girls looked horrified. Tamara did not travel well in cars at the best of times, so this was going to truly test her resolve. We sped up and down dunes, we skidded 180 degrees in the sand and sliced through the desert terrain at speeds of up to 80km/h. It was exhilaration and excitement at its finest. I glanced at the faces of Tamara, Mum and then Lara and Isla. I don't think they shared my enthusiasm. When Lara started crying, saying she felt sick, and Mum looked at me and said, 'I am going to bloody kill you,' this confirmed as much.

We had all been given a headscarf and shawl to wear to protect us from the heat and the sand. When we reached our first location the jeep came to a skidding halt, and Lara, not a moment too soon, ripped the shawl away from her mouth and hurled the contents of her breakfast all over the desert floor. 'Don't worry, Lara,' I said as I patted her on the back. 'We are only here for another 10 hours, sweetie.'

We were shown into what looked like a garage, which brought instant relief from the heat for Tamara, Mum and the girls. We were all given a cold drink, while it was explained to us how to ride the quad bikes and to stay in a convoy. The girls were too young to drive a bike themselves, so they would go on the back of mine and Tamara's. I couldn't wait to get started. We all took off, around 12 of us in the group heading off into the desert, following the lead bike. The heat from the engine between your legs added to the overall baking temperatures. Lara sat on the back of my bike and clung on around my waist as if her life depended on it. I told her to relax her grip and that she would be fine. Mum seemed to be having a few issues with her bike, though. She dropped to the very back of our convoy, and then she eventually stopped completely. One of our guides had to double back to see what the problem was.

We drove around the desert for around 20 minutes with no sign of Mum. We rode figure-of-eight circles, went up and down the dunes and followed everything the lead bike did. Eventually, Mum caught us up. Only this time, she was riding pillion with the guide who'd gone back for her. Mum's bike had packed in the moment she sat on it, so they had to tow the broken bike back to the garage. When I looked at my mum's face, she did not look amused, not even the tiniest bit.

The guide who was now riding Mum's bike, with Mum holding on for dear life, suddenly said, 'Right, who's ready? Follow me, guys.' And with that, he was gone. Woosh! His bike kicked up a cloud of sand as he floored it and took off like a bat out of hell. All I could see through the sand cloud was my 69-year-old mother on the back of the bike, which was now being driven like a MotoGP superbike across the desert, disappearing off into the distance. Oh shit, Mum's not going to be happy, I told myself.

Sure enough, she wasn't. When we all finally arrived back at the garage, she came across to me and punched me on the shoulder. 'You,' she said. 'Why did we have to bloody do this?' Neither my mum nor Tamara had enjoyed the experience. The girls looked nonplussed too, like they were trying to figure out what had just happened. I had loved it, but I kept my joy to myself, sensing it would not be well received.

After the quad biking, it was back into the jeeps to go on to our next location—lunch at the Bedouin village, the most relaxing part of the day's itinerary. In the jeep, which once more hurtled across the terrain like a rally car, Mum told me that she'd thought she was going to die on the back of the

103

quad bike. I laughed hysterically. Tamara scolded me.

'You wouldn't have died,' I said. 'It was just a bit of fast fun in the desert. I take it you won't be doing it again?'

'Definitely not,' Mum responded, before placing her head near the open window, concentrating on not being sick.

When we arrived at the village, Lara flew out of the jeep and promptly vomited in front of the whole group. She was very good at being sick at the most inopportune moments. On a family holiday to Disney World a few years earlier, we had arrived early at the gates of Magic Kingdom, so we could see the famous rope drop and be among the first guests in the park. After we'd watched a parade of dancing princesses and Mickey and Minnie, a voice over the tannoy system started the countdown to open the park, 10, 9, 8, 7, 6, 5, 4, 3, 2, 1 …

'Welcome to the Magic Kingdom, the happiest place on Earth.' No sooner had the countdown finished than Lara projectile-vomited about 2-3 feet in front of her. It went everywhere. I have never seen a crowd disperse so quickly.

Back in the desert that day in Egypt, not just Lara but my entire family were feeling sick and disorientated. A combination of the intense desert sun and the motion of being thrown around in the jeep had taken its toll. By midday, they were all done, longing to be back at the hotel. The only problem with that was that we were not due to arrive back at the hotel till 11pm that night.

None of them wanted any lunch and looked immediately for shade in which they could shelter from the sun. I was loving the whole experience but once again kept it to myself.

We got back in the jeeps after lunch. A brief stop soon followed, allowing those who wanted it an opportunity to scramble to the top of a nearby viewpoint. I raced up. Mum, Tamara and the girls stayed in the jeep, with the air conditioning cranked up to full. The dune buggies were a tad disappointing, nothing like what I thought they would be. Again, the family elected not to partake. I was the only willing and active participant from Team Stewart, for the whole day. It was a disappointing performance from my nearest and dearest. While I drove around in a buggy trying to get the thing to go over the 15mph it was clearly locked at, both Tamara and Isla had been sick. Just Mum to go, I thought, and she almost was. The day had been a complete unmitigated disaster. I loved every minute of it, but I sympathised with my family's misery.

A misery which was compounded after a completely random evening of entertainment. An evening where we watched a dancer spinning around on the spot for one whole hour and a mediocre dinner served cold. We finally got back in the jeeps for the one-hour journey back to the hotel at 10pm. The saving grace from the evening was the fact that the sun had gone down. The temperature plummeted, and we were given blankets to wrap around us. Fearing the worst for the drive back across the desert, the driver initially once more sped away, but soon slowed down, saying, 'Joke, Joke, you are all very tired.'

The following day we were once more back around the pool. Tamara, Mum and the girls were all once more in their element. I sighed and settled in on my sun-lounger. 'Anyone got anything good to read?'

I was pretty sure that I'd just had my only adventure for the holiday. Later that day, my clipboard friend wandered across to our sunbeds and asked if we wanted to do a spectacular sunset quad bike ride in the desert that night. Both Mum and Tamara said something to the degree of 'Not a cat in hell's chance,' although I'm sure Tamara said something a little bit stronger before the word 'cat'. Tamara said I could if I wanted to. I didn't need to be asked twice.

That night I was back on a bike in the desert, and the sunset was every bit as spectacular as the glossy brochure had said it would be.

Happy that I had now experienced a little bit of adrenalin on my holiday, I was completely gobsmacked and amazed at the reaction when I flippantly suggested booking a boat cruise to go snorkelling in the Red Sea, with dolphins. 'Okay,' Tamara shot back. 'Why not? It sounds fun.' I think it was possibly the mention of the word 'dolphins'. Queue the Tom Cruise movie, *Jerry Maguire*. Shut up! You had me at dolphins, you had me at dolphins.

The day we went snorkelling, Mum decided not to come, choosing instead to have a relaxing day in her room and lounging by the pool. She made the right decision. The day was once more a disaster of epic proportions.

We boarded our vessel early in the morning for what was advertised as a half-a-day, full board trip. We would be provided with drinks and snacks and a full lunch. The sea that day was not the best. Large squalls tossed the boat around with minimal effort. Only 20 minutes into the journey, and people on board began to feel queasy. A young teenage boy sitting next to me began to be sick overboard. The speed of the boat crashing through the water and the wind direction meant that whatever he had for breakfast that morning hovered in the air for a split second then came straight back into the boat, covering him and partially me.

Once again, Tamara and the girls all looked pale. One of the guides on board began walking around and offering all the passengers a travel sickness tablet. It was a bit late for that, I thought. Visions of crystal-clear, flat, calm ocean waters and swimming in and around a pod of dolphins failed to materialise. Instead, what we were given was a quick 10-minute stop, where the engine was switched off and the boat could drift. For anyone who has never experienced seasickness, believe me, it is not a very nice sensation. It's also far worse when the boat is allowed to drift. The swaying motion from side to side is enough to test the most resilient of sturdy stomachs.

The sea was an angry, foaming mess, with waves crashing all around. We were told that dolphins had been spotted in the area, and that if we took a mask and a snorkel and went into the sea, we might be able to see them. Not one person on board was prepared to risk their life by jumping overboard. There was certainly no way I was going to throw my nine- and eight-year-old daughters into the raging maelstrom that swirled below. Come on, girls, in you go, you big jessies.

When the guides on board realised no one was prepared to go in, we took off, heading to our snorkelling spot. By now, even I was starting to feel the effects of seasickness. Luckily, where we stopped thirty minutes later was in an area of sea which was a lot calmer. I told Tamara and the girls that the best place to be was in the water, rather than on a boat bobbing up and down. Unfortunately, Lara had left her swimming cap back at the hotel. She could not go in the sea without it, as she needed to keep her ears dry due to perforated eardrums. Tamara and I took it in turns going in and out of the water for the next forty minutes, while poor Lara had to stay onboard, suffering the full effect of the swaying motion. She had curled up in a foetal position on the seat, sobbing her little heart out. How she was not sick that day, I have no idea. Yep, Dad sure did know how to show the girls how to have fun.

After being served up a lunch of fish salad which no one wanted, we began to get ready for the journey back to shore. One or two of the guides onboard wandered around, taking photos of all the occupants most of the journey back, which I thought was odd. It was only when they began to

107

tout a CD for sale, full of 'all your special memories' from the day at sea, that I realised why. Every time the poor guy and his camera came anywhere near Tamara, who was laid comatose on a bench at the back of the boat, she would let him have it. 'Do I look like I want my bloody picture taken?' she would angrily say, her dark hair matted and knotted to her delicate complexion and a line of spit and sick drooling from her mouth. Terra firma could not come quick enough.

It was not one of the better days on that holiday, and yet again I spent the rest of the day and night apologising to Tamara and the girls. 'I am sorry, guys, it looked so much better in the colour brochure.'

In a way, Tamara sometimes only has herself to blame. My wife does not travel well, whether that be in a plane flying across the Atlantic, or as a passenger in a car driving down the M1 motorway. Unless she takes a sickness tablet a few hours before we set off, she always ends up feeling very queasy and unwell. The worst place imaginable to stick Tamara is in a boat. It will not end well. Yet every time we have been away on holiday together, I have always managed to get her in a boat. You would think she would learn her lesson, but she never does.

***

Before the girls came along, what was without doubt the single most catastrophic boat adventure I managed to get her to sign up to occurred on our honeymoon. That special, once in a lifetime romantic getaway of relaxation, sun, sea, sand and se—anyway, I won't get into that, but you get the idea.

We honeymooned in Thailand for three whole weeks, a few weeks after our wedding. Unfortunately, we had booked to go off-season, but we had no choice. With Tamara being a teacher, the UK summer holidays were the only time when we could get a three-week break together. It may have been the height of summer in the UK and Europe, but in Southeast Asia, this meant one thing: monsoon. On a 20-day holiday, it rained for over half of these days, but we didn't let it dampen our spirits.

We stayed in a stunning hotel resort on the island of Phuket. The Andaman sea lapped right up to our beachfront villa. It was the picture of paradise. We had a small infinity pool as part of our villa, and for the first few nights we would take a night-time stroll on the beach and then relax in our pool, gazing out at the sea and a sky full of stars. It was heavenly.

On the third night, one of the resort staff members completely ruined the tranquillity and splendour for me for the rest of my stay. Our villa, our little piece of heaven on earth, had the most amazing views from the front, looking out across the sea. Directly behind the villa was a sloping hill which was home to a banana plantation, which the member of staff went on to say was also home to king cobras. 'I'm sorry? Say what, now?'

When it comes to snakes, I am Indiana Jones. They are the creatures on this planet that I fear the most. Tell me there is a great white shark in the ocean, and I will be the first one in. But if you tell me there is the slightest prospect that I may see a snake, I completely turn to jelly. I know this fear is irrational, and I blame it squarely on an old British TV show I remember watching one Sunday evening before bed as a small boy. In an episode of *Tales of the Unexpected,* a snake had crawled into a bed in the middle of the night while the occupants were fast asleep. You saw the snake slithering and sliding its way up through the sheets and then across the body of one of the sleeping characters, before planting its fangs firmly into his shoulder. It terrified the life out of me. I have never liked our reptilian friends since.

The fact that I had now just been told that my

honeymoon hotel was home to one of the most fearsome of the creatures, the cobra, ruined everything for me. From that moment on, there were no more moonlit walks on the beach, and I would only go in our pool when it was daylight. Tamara was not bothered one iota by their presence and just spent most of the time laughing at my cowardly fear.

Apart from sharing our paradise with cobras, the other thing that eventually led us to check out early was the fact that there was no one there. I know it was off-season, but there is quiet and then there is very quiet. Our resort was very, very quiet. This only became a problem when we would go to the restaurant and bar in the evening. After three or four days of smartening ourselves up for the evening, we eventually got to the point where we decided it was pointless making the effort if it was just going to be us again in the restaurant. We had several members of staff tending to our table each night. It was complete overkill. At one stage, it felt like we were a young prince and princess, newly married, living in a royal palace, with servants for our every need.

We sat chatting one evening and decided that we wanted to see more of Thailand. We had come to Thailand to experience the Thai culture and its sights and sounds. We were too comfortable in our resort, cocooned away from real Thailand. A taxi ride into the nearby town of Patong one day convinced us to check out. That was what we wanted to see. If our resort had been heavenly peace on earth, Patong was the complete opposite. But after spending six full days and nights of peace on earth and how's your father, we were both ready for something else.

Patong was a thriving, chaotic mix of hedonism, full moon parties on the beach, ladyboys and ping-pong shows, Thai boxing fights and Irish bars, live music venues and restaurants galore. It was perfect. Because we had checked out of our hotel 14 days early, we saved ourselves a fortune. We had been paying $150 USD a night, of which every penny was worth it. In Patong, we found a backpackers' lodge for the princely sum of $10 USD a night. We checked in for the remaining 14 nights. With the money we saved, we decided to see the real Thailand. When I say the real Thailand, what I mean is the inside of an Irish pub every night, but it was still money well spent. When we were not in the Irish pub, we did book to do other things with the many ticket touts and tour guides on the sidewalks. We spent a day white-water rafting, another day elephant trekking and another day jet-skiing.

The resort had been decimated during the Boxing Day tsunami a few years earlier. There was still large-scale rebuilding taking place everywhere, with the main beachfront locations looking like they had taken the brunt of the force of the wave and resultant damage. 250 people in Patong alone were killed when the wave hit. It was all very sad. Of special poignancy was the day we went to visit a shrine that had been left as a mark of respect for the victims. It was a place that, a few days after the wave had hit, was used as somewhere to pin up a photo of your missing loved ones. It became a lost and missing noticeboard, with every picture telling a tragic story. Months and years after the tragic disaster, the locals decided to memorialise the whole area and turn it into a garden of remembrance, leaving the pictures in place. It was as beautiful and peaceful as it was tragic. There is only one other place I have been in this world where I have felt the same sense of serenity and peaceful reflection, and that is the Ground Zero memorial fountains in New York City.

When I had first trekked to Everest Base Camp seven years earlier, I had watched a screening in Kathmandu of a new recently released movie starring Leonardo DiCaprio,

The Beach. The movie was shot on location at a beach resort which was advertised as being a short boat ride from Patong. Over the past several years, thanks to the movie, it had become a tourist attraction, with people keen to see what was described as the most stunning beach location on earth.

The beach itself was in a small bay on an island chain known as the Phi Phi islands. A one-day boat tour from Patong would take you into the bay, where you could spend an hour sunbathing and walking on the now legendary beach. I was most definitely up for it. I just needed to get Tamara on board. We were on our honeymoon, so what could be better than seeing the most fantastic beach on earth? I didn't need to sell it that much. Tamara was as keen as I was to visit.

I have very rarely seen Tamara curse or lose the plot, but a few days later on our boat ride to the beach, she did both. I haven't seen a full repeat of that day since. On the rare occasion when it has reared up slightly, it has usually involved a boat and the sea. The day we sailed across to the beach, the monsoon rains were in full effect. We had to shelter under a canopy near where the boat would leave for a good 40 minutes while the heavens opened. For a while, it appeared that the trip was going to be cancelled. I could see our boat captain talking nervously to the tour guide, assuming it was about the viability of whether we should undertake the crossing or not. Once the rains had subsided, the decision to go was made.

Our boat that day was a large speedboat-type craft, with six rows of seats arranged like the ones on a plane, with an aisle down the middle. The boat's capacity was around 16 passengers. There were a few families from Europe on board with their kids, a few Americans, an Australian couple and then rather bizarrely a group of several Indian men, all suited and booted, wearing shirts and ties. I remember thinking at the time, It takes all sorts, I guess. One of the Indian chaps looked green around the gills before we had even left the port.

Our guide for the day introduced himself and went through all the safety protocols that we all needed to adhere to if we wanted to live. Yes, that's correct. The guide said that, unless we paid attention to him talking and listened to what he was saying, we could all die. What a great start. All the while he was talking, the Indian men completely ignored him and kept chatting away among themselves. I sensed that this had got his back up, as he continually glanced in their direction.

We were each given a life jacket and a bottle of water, and then the boat took off at what felt like 100mph. After launching over each wave, the boat would be airborne for a fraction of a second before coming down heavy and striking the sea with a loud thwacking sound. Tamara looked at me rather nervously. After ten more minutes of this racing across the sea, leaping over each wave and then crashing back down again with a thwack, our guide stood up in the middle to speak to us again in his broken English.

'Okay, listen up, everyone. You people listen to me, this is very important. If I say everyone to this side of the boat, then we all stand up and move across to this side. Do you understand?' He pointed to the right-hand side of the boat as he spoke.

Once again, our Indian contingency onboard blatantly disregarded everything the guide was saying and carried on chatting loudly among themselves. I wasn't sure why we all suddenly needed to move from one side of the boat to the other, but I am sure it had to do with balance and equalling out the weight in the boat in case we were about to capsize. I didn't share this with Tamara. It would only add to the rising panic levels she was already feeling. As the boat thundered through the sea, it began to rain once more. A flash of lightning lit up the darkening sky. Thwack! The boat landed back in the sea with the loudest thud so far. Some of the children on board screamed a little as it went.

As the Indians continued conversing among themselves, the rain started to come down more heavily, and we were all beginning to become soaked and cold. The guide started to tell us about the day's timings and when we would be arriving at an island for a lunch stop. There, he said, we could get off the boat and stretch our legs. We would also be given some bread to feed the fish in the shallows of the shoreline.

As he spoke and informed us of when we would reach 'the beach,' later in the day, he became angrier by the second.

'We will pull into Maya Bay at around 3.00pm and stay till 4.30pm. Is that understood?' No one responded. He tried again, this time louder. 'I said, is that understood?'

A collective muffled 'yes' went out around the boat. We were all now trying desperately to keep dry and to stop the horizontal rain from hitting our faces. Someone at the front of the boat unfastened their life jacket, took it off and held it out in front, using it as a shield to deflect the torrent of water that was firing into the boat, from both the sea and the rain. Thinking this was a great idea, we all followed suit.

'No, please, life jackets on, life jackets on. This is very dangerous; you could die if you do not listen.'

Some of the children in the boat began to cry and wail.

The guide approached the group of Indians and asked them what time our lunch stop was, and when we would arrive at the beach. When they replied that they didn't know, he completely lost it. He turned away and began to speak to everyone else, one at a time. 'You, what time do we arrive at the beach?' Three o'clock. 'Yes, correct.' He moved to the next person. 'What time do we arrive at the beach?' Three o'clock. 'Yes, good.' He asked me. 'And you. What time do we—'

I interrupted him before he could finish. '3.00pm.'

I felt like a naughty child who was about to be chastised if they got it wrong. 'Yes,' he said. He went around the entire boat, asking us all what time we would arrive. When we all gave him the same answer, he went back to the Indians. 'How is it everyone else on this boat has been listening to me and you are choosing to ignore everything I say? Please tell me.' The chap who, earlier that morning, I thought had looked a little off-colour shrugged his shoulders and held his hands to his face. A second later, he stood up and vomited into the aisle, wiped his mouth and sat back down.

For the next 40 minutes, we held our life jackets out in front of us to stop the deluge of water, while the boat continued to surge through the sea, crashing down off every wave. The Indian chap's sick sloshed up and down the aisle. The smell was nauseating. A German woman also threw up, followed by one of the kids on the boat. I had never felt so sick in all my life, but I managed to refrain from adding to the concoction that was steadily building on the floor of the boat.

If the boat did capsize, we would all have been done for. We all had life jackets, but not one of them was being used as it was intended to be used. Throughout the whole ordeal, Tamara had kept her head buried between her knees. She looked up only once, to speak. 'I hate you,' she told me before putting her head back down.

The storms couldn't last, and eventually the rain stopped, and the sea became calmer. We were going to survive. Despite our guide telling us we may die, none of us had.

This was a relief. Dying would have certainly ruined the honeymoon. A few of us began to high-five one another.

The boat slowed into a sheltered harbour on a remote island. It was a relief to get onto dry land. We stopped for an hour, which we all needed to recover from the ordeal. A little straw shack was selling ice-cold drinks and ice lollies. An orange ice lolly and a bottle of Sprite had never tasted so good. After feeding the fish with the bread we had been given, we were once more back in the boat, which by now had been cleaned down. We were finally on our way to the beach. All was back to being well with the world.

All was well for the next 90 minutes. The sea was much calmer, and the rain stayed away. We had clear blue skies for the rest of the day. When we were half an hour from reaching our destination, our guide stood up to speak to us.

'I am afraid I have some bad news. We are not going to be able to visit Maya Bay. There are too many boats, and conditions are very dangerous.'

One of the Indians sarcastically said, 'Are we all going to die again?'

Then they started laughing. Neither I nor anyone else on the boat saw the funny side.

'No,' our guide continued. 'There are strong currents, sharp rocks under the ocean and lots of people all trying to cross a rope ladder. It is too dangerous.'

Tamara suddenly looked up, as if she had just become aware of what was being said.

'Hang on,' she said, with anger in her voice. 'Are you telling me that I can't go to see the beach?'

'Yes, Madam, this is what I am saying. It is very dangerous.'

The veins in Tamara's temple began to throb. I could see the anger rising from within. And then it happened. She completely lost her shit.

'The only reason this idiot got me on this boat this morning,' she shouted, emphasizing the word 'idiot' as she looked directly at me, 'was so we could go to see this beach from that movie, and you are now telling me, after everything that has happened on this goddamn boat, that we aren't even going to do that?'

She was becoming more incensed as she spoke. The guide started to speak, but Tamara cut him dead. 'You have got to be fucking kidding me!'

A silence descended across the boat. But he wasn't kidding. We never got to see the beach. Tamara had only said what everyone else, except for the minors on board, had been thinking.

Granted, on that honeymoon in Thailand we never did get to see that famous beach, but on the flip side, we had an amazing adventure. It was action-packed, and other than the day at sea in that boat, we had the best of times. The six days in the cobra-infested paradise at the start of the honeymoon had even resulted in a lot more than we had bargained for. A month or so after being home, a test confirmed that Tamara was pregnant with Lara, our lasting gift from Thailand.

***

I have seen some amazing things in my 47 years on this earth. I have been to some incredible places and witnessed incredible things. Other than the places I have travelled to that have involved my mountain adventures, such as Nepal, Tibet and Argentina, nearly everywhere else has been with my family.

In late December 2016, a month after my Everest book had been released, Tamara surprised me with a gift. It was to say 'well done' on writing and publishing my story. On a Black Friday deal, she had booked return flights and accommodation for three nights in Reykjavik in Iceland, for all four of us and my mum.

She knew that one of my bucket list items had always been to see to the northern lights. December is one of the best times to see them, and Iceland was one of the best places to see them from. We flew from Edinburgh, stopping off at the world-famous Christmas market on the way. Once in Iceland, I arranged to hire a car. This seemed to be the best way to travel around the country, which essentially had one main ring road.

The main tourist attraction was a tour called the Golden Circle. This consisted of three stunning locations, all in the southwest of the country: a national park called Thingvellir, which was the meeting location of the Eurasian and North American tectonic plates; a large geyser, similar to what you might see at Yellowstone in the US; and Gullfoss, one of the country's most spectacular waterfalls. The whole tour could easily be done in one day, providing you had transport. Bus tour operators charged an extortionate price, but you could self-drive the route in just over three hours, so that's what we decided to do.

Reykjavik, the capital city, was compact, cute and curious. Those three Cs is how I have described it ever since to anyone who has asked. I would add a fourth to that list too: criminally expensive. I haven't been anywhere else on this planet that has been as expensive as Iceland was. Wandering around the downtown part of Reykjavik one day, we stumbled into a coffee shop, mainly to get warm from the freezing temperatures outside. Iceland in winter very rarely gets much above 3 degrees Celsius; that's 36F, for all my American friends.

We ordered two coffees, a bottle of Dr Pepper, and a chocolate crepe each for the girls. The bill came to 6,200 Icelandic Krona, which was around £36. I was gobsmacked.

Realising we would need to be careful, we found a local

supermarket and purchased some teabags, breakfast cereals and milk for mornings and a few frozen pizzas for the evenings. In the UK, this would have cost less than £10. In Iceland, it cost £25.

Nowhere sold alcohol, so we saved money on that. There are strict rules on buying alcohol in Iceland. It is heavily taxed, and prices are astronomical. As a result, supermarkets are not allowed to sell it. Tamara was not happy. After all, wine is to women what duct tape is to us men. It fixes everything.

The day we drove the Golden Circle was spectacular. Winter daylight was short in Iceland, so we had a race against time to see all three of the main attractions on the tour. It began to snow in the morning and did not let up for the whole day. We had our very own picture-perfect winter wonderland.

The steps down to Thingvellir were covered in ice by the time we arrived, which Isla, my youngest, discovered as she went skidding on her back from top to bottom. Back in the car, and a 50-minute drive brought us to Strokkur, the geyser. The girls loved this natural geothermal phenomenon, and we easily spent an hour watching water being thrown 20 to 40 metres into the air every 10 minutes or so.

Back in the car again, and before we would reach the last destination, the Gullfoss waterfall, we pulled off the road at what looked like a service station. We needed to eat. Once again, I was left open-mouthed at the prices. We decided to let the girls eat and ordered them both a burger and fries. When the cashier gave me the bill, I felt like asking her how she slept at night, but I resisted.

The waterfall was spectacular under a full frozen winter coat. It was simply breath-taking. We arrived just in time before the visitor centre closed for the day. The snow continued to come down, and a thick crust of ice covered the walkways and paths down to the waterfall itself. One of these walkways took you down close to the edge of the falls, where you could feel the water splashing back on your face. With only 30 minutes before the centre closed, it appeared all the tourists were keen to do just that.

It looked to be a steep 15-minute descent down to the waterfall, on treacherous paths. I decided we didn't have time, plus I had Mum to think about. I didn't want her breaking something slipping over on the ice. We stayed at the top and decided to play a game of guessing who would slip over on the walkway. It was great fun. 'That lady in the white coat and black hat. She's definitely going to slip over.' Sure enough, a few seconds later, we would be in fits of laughter at the poor unfortunate lady having to pick herself up from an incredibly slippery, icy walkway. Sometimes, other people's misfortune can be another person's entertainment. We spent 10 minutes playing this game, in fits of laughter the whole time. I hoped I wouldn't go to hell for suggesting it.

By now we had been in Iceland two full days and had not seen the northern lights, the main reason we had come. That night was to be the night. The lights hadn't been seen for about a week, but the signs were good that tonight there would be a strong chance. High geomagnetic activity had been detected on the KP index; a system used to measure the aurora's strength. According to this index, tonight was a 2-3 on the scale, which meant moderate activity with good chances of catching the lights if you left the light pollution of Reykjavik. We were up for that, so after dinner of frozen pizza again, we hit the road in search of the lights. We drove around for two hours, driving to all the locations we had been told to visit. But the lights stubbornly refused to appear. The girls were beginning to become fractious and bored in the back of the car, so after another half an hour of driving through some of Iceland's back roads, we decided to call it a night. To say I was disappointed was an understatement. It was like going to Nepal to see Everest, but the mountain remains hidden behind a blanket of clouds the whole time you're there.

Back in our apartment in the city, I knew Tamara was especially disappointed, as I think deep down, she really thought we would have a good chance of seeing them. That was why we had come to Iceland in late December, the best time of year to see them. If we could have got our money back, I am sure we would have done. We all felt cheated. With our limited amount of time, it was never a guarantee, but we had given ourselves the best opportunity within that short timescale to see this celestial spectacular. Sadly, it was not meant to be.

At 3.00am, we were all cosy in our beds, fast asleep, when Tamara switched on the lights to the apartment. 'Wake up, wake up, sleepy heads,' she shouted. Wondering what was going on, I stuck my head out of the duvet. 'The alert level has gone up,' she said. 'We might see the lights.' In Iceland, it didn't matter whether it was early morning, late afternoon or night. If it was dark, there was a chance. I weighed up our options. Get up, get dressed, get the girls up and then get back in the car and drive around the city's backroads again in the hope that we might see them. Or stay in my warm bed and go back to sleep. I looked at my mum and then at the girls, who looked very reluctant to get up.

'You guys can go,' I said. 'But I'm staying in bed.' I turned over and pulled the duvet tighter around my neck.

Tamara was livid. 'I can't believe you. We've come to Iceland to see the northern lights, and now we have a great opportunity to see the lights, and you'd rather stay in bed.'

She had a point, but I stubbornly refused to get out of

121

bed. If it were 100 percent guaranteed that we would see them, then I would have been the first one up and ready, but I didn't think it was going to happen.

Tamara, Mum and the girls got up, got dressed and left the apartment. Tamara slammed the door behind her. I lay in my bed for another 20 minutes or so with guilt sweeping over me like a rapid hot flush. 'Fuck it!' I shouted, before dragging my backside out of bed, brushing my teeth, getting ready and then going out into the early morning freeze. I caught up with Tamara, Mum and the girls browsing around a 24-hour shop just up the road. It wasn't even 4.00am. We got back in the car and did go for a short drive to where it was suggested we may see the lights, but guess what? No lights. Be that as it may, I remained in the doghouse for the rest of the day.

On the last full day and night, we crammed in as much as possible. We visited the great northern lights exhibition in downtown Reykjavik. This was not as great as it sounded. It was a small visitor attraction which, using multimedia displays, told you about the history and science behind the lights and how they are formed. There was, however, a room which was similar to a planetarium. You sat back in your seat and looked up to see a projection of the Aurora Borealis in full effect, dancing across the ceiling. I took a photo on my phone and uploaded it to Instagram with the following caption: 'In Iceland, seeing the northern lights. Truly amazing.' A few comments appeared, saying things like 'Wow' and 'Really jealous'. If only they knew the truth. #northernlightsmyarse #fullofshit #fake

Before we departed back to the UK, there was one place we all wanted to visit. It was the one thing we had identified as being the highlight of the trip, other than seeing the lights. It was a tourist attraction called The Blue Lagoon. It was the country's premier tourist attraction and even referred to itself on its impressive, snazzy-looking website as one of the 25 top wonders of the world. Discover the waters of the blue lagoon, it also stated, and journey through a spa of the volcanic earth and harmonize with nature.

The girls were busting to harmonize with nature, so we had to go and see for ourselves. Tamara and I had deliberately saved the best till last.

The lagoon was a geothermal spa, just outside of Reykjavik. The spa was supplied by water used in a nearby geothermal power station and consisted of a series of natural outdoor pools and spas with a water temperature constantly between 37 – 39 degrees Celsius. It looked and sounded incredible. What better way to spend your last day visiting a new country than to simply kick back and relax.

We hadn't booked (luckily), as we weren't sure which day to attend. Plus, I knew we could pay on the door. For a three-hour visit, it was going to cost around 30,000 Icelandic Krona for all five of us. That was over £170 in pound sterling. To visit a swimming pool. Yes, okay, I know it was more than just a swimming pool, but I still could not get over how expensive it was. It was the story of the whole three days in Iceland, and unfortunately, it was a case of when in Rome. We had planned to go later in the day when it got dark. I figured that it would add a level of magic to the experience, being outside in a hot pool at night. I thought to myself that it might even snow, and how utterly cool would that be?

Before we left, we had a bite to eat in the communal cafeteria that was part of our apartment complex. The girl who brought us over our hot drinks and snacks took an interest when we were looking at the brochure for the lagoon.

'Are you planning on going there?' she enquired.

'Yes, we are. We're going as soon as we leave here,' I responded.

'Can I be honest with you? she asked. 'I wouldn't go there if I were you. It's rubbish and overpriced.'

I remember instantly thinking, Oh, great. The one thing we have all been looking forward to, destroyed in two seconds flat. However, all was not lost. The girl carried on telling us about another place, which was a lot closer in the city. She said it was mainly used by locals, and not many tourists had even heard of it. She was right. I had never been told about it. I think, perhaps, the Icelandic government wanted to keep earning taxes from its premier tourism jewel in the crown. She strongly recommended that we went to this other place instead. It sounded almost identical to everything we could experience at The Blue Lagoon, but for a fraction of the price and with less lavishness and luxury. I was on board the second she said, 'a fraction of the price.' Screw luxury. Price wins every time.

Following the directions my new best friend had provided, we found the place easily. It was most definitely off the beaten path and away from the tourist areas of the city. The girls were a tad disappointed we were no longer going to visit the lagoon, but at the end of the day, if this place had a pool, they would be happy.

My first impression was one of disappointment. The building itself reminded me of a UK 1960s-built, council-owned leisure centre. It looked a bit worn out. But you know what they say about never judging a book by its cover. That was certainly the case with this place. Once inside, we paid almost £7 for admission. Yes, that was £7. And not each. That was for all of us. God bless coffee attendants. Once through the turnstile, we then had to separate. Tamara, Mum and the girls headed for the ladies' changing area while I went to the men's.

I had to strip naked and shower thoroughly before putting on my board shorts and being allowed into the main area of pools outdoors. This was so the natural waters of the pool could remain as clean and pollutant-free as possible. It was a shared shower, which meant I shared my naked wash with several burly, bearded, Viking-looking chaps. I had a short conversation with one of them, who continued to lather up and wash his tackle the entire time we spoke. 'Ha Ha,' he said. 'We beat the mighty English in football.' He was referring to the recent Euro football tournament, where indeed he was right. Iceland had beaten England 2-1.

Once I was outdoors, I waited for the girls to emerge. Lara and Isla both looked ready to die of embarrassment. Tamara explained that the naked shower wash had taken them all by surprise. The girls didn't know where to look. There were bouncing, lathered boobs everywhere. For a split moment, I couldn't help but think how wonderful a unisex shower would have been, but then snapped myself out of it. Stop it, Ellis. You're with your wife, daughters and Mum, for goodness' sake. Hey, you can still window shop. It doesn't mean you're going to buy.

The place was amazing. It was a secret nirvana, away from the main tourists. The hot geothermal spas ranged in temperature from 37 degrees through to a scorching 46 degrees Celsius. There was even an ice plunge pool, which I could not bring myself to brave. Every one of us loved every moment of it. We stayed for a couple of hours, relaxing and enjoying the ambience. There was a pool for the girls to play water polo in, and an outside bar selling refreshments and soft drinks. As I lay back in one of the pools, staring up at the heavens, I felt something wet and cold land on my nose, then another, and then another. It had started to snow. The snow came down heavily for

125

the rest of our stay. It was simply magical. Not seeing the northern lights a day earlier had been a big down. This, right now, was most definitely an up. I soaked up every moment of it, not wanting it to end. It was the highlight of our entire trip to Iceland. Tamara looked at me and kissed me. 'I love you,' she said. I was finally forgiven.

I haven't travelled the world, but I feel very privileged and blessed to have been where I have been and seen what I have seen. I have done it all on the backdrop of not being wealthy. Misadventure has abounded at every opportunity, but it has been a complete joy.

I have driven the great ocean road on Australia's southern coast, cuddling a koala bear in the process. I have been massaged by an elephant in Thailand, got drunk in Dublin with an American Airlines captain on whiskey and rum.

I have been on the guest list to see a Grammy award-winning band in New York City, all because Tamara showed the drummer how to use Snapchat in a pizza café, and I have been taught how to dance the tango on the streets of Buenos Aires.

I have cruised slowly down South Beach, Miami in my 5.0. Okay, so I was with Tamara, the girls and my mum, plus it was a rental. But it still counts.

I have stared a great white shark in the eyes from less than 2cm away and not flinched. The fact that it was suspended in a tank, dead and preserved doesn't matter. It's the experience that counts.

I have climbed the highest mountain in South America, sleeping out under the stars, gazing at the Southern Cross, wondering what it's all about. I have attempted to climb the highest mountain in the world, twice.

I have dined in one of the finest restaurants in the world in Hong Kong, and I crossed the border into China for the day, just to buy some counterfeit DVDs. I have gambled in casinos in Macau with Chinese businessmen and lost. I have taken my young daughters to see a newly born panda bear, then realised they were more popular than the newly born bear.

I have shared a hot tub with the British band Take That (true story) and had a thousand-people chanting my name at a German beer festival in Stuttgart (another true story).

I could go on. Perhaps I will save it and some of the above encounters for another book one day.

All these experiences have left footsteps in my heart. It is correct what they say, travel most definitely broadens the mind. Out of everywhere I have ever been, everything I have ever done and every adventure, misadventure and place and culture I have embraced, nothing comes close to those experiences I have had with my family by my side.

You know what they say. 'A family that travels together stays together.' I would not change a single thing. Well, perhaps I should stop insisting on boat trips and maybe I should have got out of bed that morning to go and find those northern lights. One day.

CHAPTER FIVE
MY REAL LIFE HEROES

'Only a life lived for others is a life worth living.'
Albert Einstein

Whoever said you should never meet your heroes as you will only be disappointed clearly doesn't know some of mine. Generally, I have always done what I have wanted to do and been who I want to be. I am rarely influenced or inspired by another individual, but that's not to say I am not. There have been several people who have affected the course of my life, mostly in a positive way, while some ... well, not so much.

Before I speak about some of those who have inspired me along this journey of life, here is a little list of those who haven't. In no order, I don't like:

- The Child Catcher from *Chitty Chitty Bang Bang*
- Pazuzu, the demon from *The Exorcist*
- Sergeant Dillon (See Chapter One, 'Growing Pains'. Another individual who, along with the Child Catcher, was responsible for ruining my childhood.)
- My old maths teacher, who one day took a metre ruler and gave me twenty whacks across my hands.

That's it. My list of people who have left mental scarring on my very fragile psyche. I am a very tolerant person for the most part, and I always look for the good in people. I like to believe that more people are good than bad. Jack Johnson, the American singer/songwriter, even wanted to know where all the good people had gone, in his 2005 song 'Good People'. They are right there, Jack. They haven't gone anywhere. You just need to know where to look to find them.

Goodness, positivity, and kindness are all around us. If you cannot find it, you need to open your eyes slightly wider. Some of the more notable people who have left their lasting influence on my life include:

- Dave Price, my old dragon boat coach

- Muhammad Ali

- Luke Skywalker

- Doug Scott (obviously)

- Danger Mouse

- Tara, a girl who was in the year above me at secondary school

I am lucky to know and to have personally known three people on this list. The bottom one I got to know very well one night when I turned 15. I wish I could say that I had met Mark Hamill, but that was never going to happen. Dave and Doug more than made up for it, mind. Ironically, meeting Muhammad Ali is not as far-fetched as it sounds. There is a connection to the great man, and it involved my wife Tamara.

Several years ago, I had gone along to one of Tamara's staff Christmas parties, at an old school where she previously worked. We were sitting at a table that included the school principal and some other senior leaders. Late in the night, with the drink flowing, Ken, the principal, began a game that went around the table about who the most famous person you had ever met was. The winner as decided by everyone present would get a prize. Everyone then offered up their most famous encounters, accompanied by a short anecdote about how they'd met. Tamara couldn't think of anyone, so she was skipped. I answered that I had once knocked a pint of Guinness out of the hand of Gary Pallister, an ex-England and Manchester United footballer. He tried to catch it, which made things worse, as he then proceeded in covering himself in the black stuff. True story. I offered to buy him a new pint, which he accepted. It's a good job I didn't need to replace the gleaming, crisp white shirt he had on. It was probably very expensive.

As the game progressed, the rest of the guests around the table offered up their entries. We had a John Major and also The Krankies, a Scottish comedy duo who appeared on TV in the '80s; The Green Cross Code Man, who was a costumed superhero created in England in the '70s to teach young children how to cross a road safely. Kylie Minogue; David Beckham, which elicited some positive reactions; the band Steps; and then finally Jimmy Saville, which silenced the table and killed the conversation quickly. Ken, the principal, broke the silence.

'Come on, Tamara, back to you. Who is the most famous person you have met? There must be someone.'

Her answer has stayed with me to this day. 'I met Muhammad Ali once.' she said. 'Does that count?'

The table erupted in complete shock, euphoria and gasps as a spray of alcoholic mist from everyone's mouths covered the table. 'What?' Ken shouted across the table, in complete shock that Tamara hadn't thought to mention this

131

the first time around.

Unbelievably, she wasn't lying. She had met the boxer known around the world as the greatest of all time when she was around 10 years old. Back then, Tamara and her family lived in Saudi Arabia, due to her father's work as a doctor. One day, Tamara was playing outside the compound where she was living when Ali strode past. She had no idea who he was but could see he must have been important, as lots of people swarmed around him. Tamara and her sister managed not only to speak to him for a few moments, but also to get his autograph, which she later lost.

Tamara was awarded the bottle of bubbly.

Doug.

The first time I met someone from my list who had been an inspiration of mine, I was in my early 20s. I attended a slideshow talk given by Doug Scott at the local town hall. I didn't meet him per se, but I sat in the audience, mesmerised by his tales of adventure and sometimes misadventure. Doug, as the first Brit to summit Everest, had been an inspiring figure to me growing up.

The next time our paths would cross was in November 2015, several months after I came home from Everest. Ironically, it was in the same venue where I'd seen him speak the first time. This time, Doug was there raising money for his charity, 'Community Action Nepal', or CAN, as it's more commonly known. He presented a talk and short film about his 1975 ascent of the south-west face of Everest, in which he became the first Brit to reach the top of the mountain, alongside Dougal Haston. That year would mark the 40th anniversary of that ascent. This time I stayed back and bought a signed copy of a new book he had just released called Up and About: The Hard Road to Everest, which I think is a brilliant title for a book. I even got a photo next to the great man, holding his book. I was completely made up.

Also in the audience that night were the brother and sister to the late Joe Tasker, a British mountaineer who had often climbed with Doug. Sadly, Joe was killed on Everest in 1982. He was a prolific climber who hailed from Billingham, a small town up the road. I was introduced to Joe's sister and brother and said what an honour it was to meet the family of such an esteemed and legendary mountaineer. It was. I am always in awe of what the pioneering British mountaineers from the '60s and '70s achieved. They helped to solidify Britain's reputation as being home to some of the finest climbers the world had ever seen, which Doug Scott was, of course, part of.

It was this evening that gave me the idea of making my book launch a year later a charitable occasion, donating the proceeds from the night to Doug and CAN.

I wouldn't see Doug again until after my book launch evening. But the day we finally did meet up will stay with me for a long time to come. It was December 1st, a few weeks after the book launch. I had over £3,000 to give to Doug and CAN, the combined totals raised from the evening. I had contacted the CAN office by email a week earlier to ask for bank details to transfer the money, but they said it would be much nicer if I came to Doug's house instead, where he could thank me personally.

Doug's cottage nestled at the bottom of Carrock Fell, in a small hamlet in the Lake District called Hesket Newmarket. This was a couple of hours' drive from my home in Teesside. I travelled across that day with my friend Andrew, who had been instrumental in the book launch evening. He was as much a part of the success of the evening as I was, possibly more so. I figured it would be nice for Andrew to properly meet Doug too. We also packed our walking gear so we could go up nearby Carrock Fell after our meeting. The plan was to do the polite British thing of 'having a cup of tea and some biscuits', give Doug the cheque and be on our way, off up the hills. Doug had other ideas, though.

I had prepared a short speech in my head, during the car journey over the Pennines, of what I wanted to say. This was how much of an honour it was to present him with the cheque, and that he was a real hero to me. I also wanted to give him one of my books, which was completely off-the-charts insane. Doug was a living mountaineering superstar, who had been the first person from these shores to reach the top of the highest mountain on the planet. Did I think he would want to read my story of attempting to do a fraction of what he had done in his life? No, probably not. But it still wasn't going to stop me from asking. He could use the book as a door wedge, for all I cared, if he accepted it.

'Hi Doug, how's it going?' I said when we were brought through into what looked like the working offices for CAN. CAN had provided us with a car boot full of Nepalese trinkets and signed prints to sell or advertise at my book launch. We had arranged to pick it all up from Darlington Civic Theatre, where Doug was giving a talk a week before our evening was due to take place. Andrew drove across one night and collected it all. That day, we were returning what we hadn't sold.

We did manage to auction off several of the prints, which raised several hundred pounds towards the total money raised. There was one print that I specifically wanted myself, but unfortunately, the MD of Cameron's Brewery outbid me on the night. It was a photo taken by Doug of Dougal Haston climbing through the Khumbu Icefall on Everest. It was signed by Doug and Chris Bonington, the expedition leader. It was a stunning atmospheric image, and I had visions of it adorning the walls of my living room. It also had special meaning for me, as the Icefall was as far as I'd got on my own Everest quest.

'Doug, that image of the Icefall that we sold was simply sublime. If you ever print it again, please let me know, as I lost out on the night and I was gutted,' I said as Doug began to chase a little dog around his office.

'Eh, get here, no. Eh, you little bugger, I said here.' The dog, which looked long in the tooth, was paying no attention to Doug whatsoever. 'I've got another one here if you'd like it, youth,' Doug offered.

'Yes, please,' I rather enthusiastically responded. For a moment, I thought he was giving me a print for free, as a way of saying thanks for the cheque we were about to present to him, but Doug had spotted an opportunity to up the total.

'These prints usually auction for around £200, but I'll let you have one for ... let's say £195?'

Cursing my negotiation skills, or lack of, I agreed. To be honest, I would have paid £300, I loved the print that much.

Before we were about to leave and head up the fell that day, Doug looked down at Andrew's feet and then at mine, before saying to us both, 'What size foot are you, fellas?' After we both told him, he told us to follow him out into his garden.

He walked us to the very bottom of his garden, all the while trying to get his disobedient dog to do as he said. 'Here, here, here, I said. No, not over there. Here.'

The dog was blatantly ignoring its master's requests to heel. If dogs could talk, I am sure this one would have been saying, 'Fuck you, I'll do whatever I goddamn like.' It didn't stop Doug from trying, though.

At the bottom of the garden, Doug unlocked a double door into a large shed. From floor to ceiling there were dozens and dozens of pairs of walking boots. They all looked brand new, too. Doug informed us they were all minor cosmetic seconds from the Italian boot manufacturer Scarpa. They sent Doug all the boots that failed quality control. Doug would then arrange for them to be sent out to Nepal, where they would be given out to the local village people in the Himalayas.

'Help yourselves, fellas,' Doug said. He told us that if we could find a few pairs in our size, we were welcome to keep them. It looked as though it would be like trying to find a needle in a haystack, but we gave it a go.

'That's very kind, thanks,' we both said.

'No problem. But while you're looking, you wouldn't mind tidying and sorting them all out for me, would you?'

Doug informed us that all the right boots had been separated from the lefts and that the whole shed was one huge mess which needed sorting. 'If you find the right and left of a particular pair, just tie the laces together,' he added, before heading back to the house, all the while calling out after his defiant little mutt.

I looked at Andrew, incredulous at what we had both just been asked to do, then I burst out laughing. Andrew followed suit. 'Are you okay with this?' I asked.

'Yeah. It's not every day you get asked to tidy the boot shed of the first Brit to summit Everest,' he said with a wry smile.

We spent around two hours in the shed that day on our hands and knees, matching lefts to rights. Once we had finished, we went back up the house, each clutching several pairs of Scarpa footwear, which Doug said we could have for our efforts.

Even though we had spent longer at Doug's cottage than I would have liked, we still had time to hike up nearby Carrock Fell before it turned dark, which was under a full blanket of crisp winter snow. Before we left, I gave Doug a copy of my book and asked him if he'd mind if I took a photo of him holding it, to which he kindly agreed. He asked me if the book included my background and my story of what made me want to go to Everest. When I said that it did, he said, 'I'll probably give it a go, then. I'm not interested in the Everest parts, but I like to read about people's real lives.'

That made perfect sense to me, as I had always thought, when seeing Doug give a talk, that he spoke about the mountain very nonchalantly. When I had gone to his talk a year earlier on his ascent of the south-west face of Everest, he'd spent the first 10 minutes talking about CAN and some other trips he had done, before he finally said, 'So I had best talk about Everest, seeing as how that's why you're all here.' I genuinely got the impression that he would rather have spoken about pretty much anything else. He was the most remarkably modest and unassuming man I have ever met, before and since. He had achieved incredible feats in his heyday as a climber, but you wouldn't have realised, spending time in his company.

That day in his cottage, tidying his boots, was the last day I saw Doug Scott, but I often recounted the story of the time I spent a day in Doug's shed in my public talks. It always goes down well and raises a chuckle, much in part, I think, to the affection with which Doug is held by the British public. The photo that I got that day of Doug posing with my book at his cottage meant the world to me. I have two photos side by side in a frame in my study at home. I am standing next to Doug in both. In one, I am holding a copy of his book, and in the other, he is holding mine.

I will always remember that day at Doug's cottage, tidying walking boots in a shed, while Doug chased his defiant dog around the garden. It's not every day you can say to yourself that you got to spend a day in the presence of one of your real-life heroes. That's just how I roll, I guess.

Tony.

Often, the individuals who go on to inspire and leave their mark on me are not famous people in the limelight. They are generally everyday folk, like you and me. I have found in my life that it's those all around us who have the capacity to inspire and motivate. You don't need to look to the silver screen, the football field or an athletics track to find modern-day heroes. They could be sitting right next to you on the bus or standing behind you in the queue at Starbucks. Heroes can be found everywhere. Sometimes you find them, other times they find you.

As a small boy, Tony loved to pore over maps. He would also love nothing more than to read, hour after hour, old copies of National Geographic magazine. Tony had a deep interest in the mountain ranges of the world, and in particular, Everest. He dreamed of one day standing on the mountain's summit. After graduating from university with a degree in Geography, Tony put his backpack on and travelled around Europe. A few years later, aged 24, he visited Nepal for the first time, which reaffirmed his love of mountains, although he didn't see Everest on this trip. After several years working in the rail industry, he began to get restless and was able to leave work under a voluntary redundancy scheme. This allowed him to backpack his way around the world for four months with a friend. Tony returned home for two months, but again the lure of travel and adventure were calling his name. This time he solo backpacked, with plans of seeing the world. But on his travels, he fell in love with Indonesia and decided to stay. He took a job teaching English in Jakarta. It was here that Tony then met and fell in love with Rini, who came from a small town near Java.

Tony and Rini married and spent the next several years living in Indonesia, where Tony continued to teach. In 2002, Tony and Rini moved back to the UK and settled in Worcester. Tony took a post teaching English to adult language students. Everything was working out well. They had both tried for a family for some years, with no luck. Then one day the opportunity to try I.V.F treatment came their way. After just one course of treatment, all their hopes and dreams came true when it was confirmed that Rini was pregnant. Not only that, but they were expecting triplets. Everything went well until the 23rd week, when Rini spent four days in hospital after going into early labour. Knowing that the chance of a baby surviving at 24 weeks was slim, their entire world imploded around them. The chance of triplets surviving such an early stage was even less. They were presented with the brutal and honest reality that, even if any of their babies survived, they would have to face up to the possibility that the babies may have significant disabilities.

Be that as it may, Jewel was born first, weighing just 630g. Two days later, Milla and Louisa joined their sister. Jewel sadly only lived for 17 days. Milla and Louisa spent five months in hospital fighting infection and setbacks. Both girls had operations to repair their sight. Unfortunately, the surgeon was not able to save the sight in Louisa's left eye. Louisa also had to have an operation to repair a hole in her heart.

Eventually, the girls battled through and were able to go home with their mum and dad, but this was just the start of the fight. After one year of having the girls home, a routine appointment at a hospital in Worcester confirmed what both Tony and Rini had suspected. There was something not right about Milla. She was diagnosed with cerebral palsy. If she couldn't walk or stand within a year, she never would.

She never did. Milla was confined to a wheelchair for the rest of her life, with spastic quadriplegia. After another year, she would also have an operation to have a stomach feeding tube fitted. Despite all this, Milla was a happy little girl, always smiling.

Things began to take their toll on both Mum and Dad. Tony became exhausted from teaching full time and caring for his daughters. Life was a constant pattern of sleepless nights, hospitalisations for the girls, operations, appointments and caring for a severely disabled daughter 24 hours a day. Tony was at the end of his tether. With no family support in Worcester and Rini's family in Indonesia, they had no one to turn to for help. Life was incredibly tough.

To avoid the crippling effects of depression, Tony began to busy himself with fundraising challenges. Just a year after the girls were born, he began raising money for charities for premature and sick babies by taking part in endurance cycling events. Many challenges followed over the next few years, including climbing Kilimanjaro, cycling from Worcester to London and back in two days and Worcester to Dublin in six.

In 2012, Tony finally achieved a boyhood dream when he trekked to Mount Everest Base Camp, raising thousands of pounds for Scope, the disability charity. Later that same year, Make A Wish UK sent Tony, Rini and the two girls to Disney World in Florida with full VIP treatment. Tony carried on with his challenges, and inspired by the work of Make A Wish, he ran the London Marathon and cycled from Land's End to John O'Groats. Life carried on this way for four more years.

Because Rini's family lived in Indonesia, visiting them

frequently proved to be difficult and expensive. When they did go to visit, it tended to be for up to six weeks at a time every couple of years. Tony would take unpaid leave from his teaching job. One such year occurred in 2016, when Tony and Rini took Louisa and Milla for a visit back to Indonesia. Ten days into the trip, Milla took ill. Mum and Dad suspected a chest infection, something they had treated many times previously. But something was different this time. Within just three days, Milla's condition had alarmingly and rapidly deteriorated. They took her to a local hospital, where she was given an inhaler to help her lungs, before she was discharged. The following morning, Tony discovered his daughter unresponsive and listless. Rini rushed Milla back to the hospital while Tony stayed with Louisa.

A few days later, Milla passed away. She had died from an overwhelming infection which led to sepsis. She was just 10 years old. As was customary in Indonesia, Milla was buried next to her grandfather. For Tony, the devastation was complete and all-encompassing. They had left for Indonesia as a family of four. They returned as three, to their home with an empty wheelchair.

Regular bereavement counselling followed. Tony had always sought solace in his teaching. He'd never felt stressed or anxious in the classroom. It was his time to shut out the outside world. Tony had suffered from his mental health before Milla's passing. Afterwards, it was debilitating. He tried desperately to ward off its crushing effects by throwing himself headfirst into further fundraising challenges. Long-distance cycle rides and 30 miles-plus day walks filled his spare time, but the depression just would not loosen its grip. He began to avoid social contact. Negativity began to overpower the positivity. Tony felt useless. His weight increased, and his self-confidence decreased with it. He stopped teaching, took an extended leave of absence and began taking anti-depressants.

When the global pandemic hit in 2020, the school where Tony had taught English to adults closed for good. All international students went home, and no one came as the world went into lockdown.

Louisa, Tony's surviving daughter, became his rock. Although being completely blind in her left eye and partially sighted in the other, she wanted to raise money in the memory of her sister Milla. She has since walked 2 miles around Worcester Racecourse and climbed 4 miles to the summit of Worcestershire Beacon, the highest point of the Malvern hills. All this from a little girl who did not take her first steps until she was four and suffers from stability issues due to her blindness.

After losing Milla, Tony took up poetry and used it as an outlet to express his emotions. He has subsequently written and published nine collections and has recently just completed his first novel. The poem at the very front of this book, *We Are Mountains*, was written for me by Tony after we became friends. If you go back and read it again, you will perhaps understand a little more of the meaning behind it now.

I didn't know Tony or his story before April 2018, but all that changed after Tony shared a tweet about how much he had been inspired by and motivated by my Everest book. I naturally responded, as I do to anyone who takes time to publicly show appreciation towards me or my book. He responded with the story you have just read. In the time since I have known Tony, I have discovered him to be one of the kindest, most compassionate and giving people I know. He battles to beat his mental health afflictions every day, and he is not afraid to admit as much through the poetry he writes and the challenges he still undertakes.

He most recently completed a 24-hour guitar playing

singalong, raising further funds for Acorns, a children's hospice which cared for Milla. His positive outlook, from a background of such heartache, has been a shining light, especially through the global pandemic and lockdown.

Whenever I am having a bad day now or feeling sorry for myself, which I do from time to time, I think of Tony and all he has been through, and then my problems pale into insignificance by comparison. This, to me, is the true definition of a hero. Someone who can impact on your life in a meaningful and positive way. Tony does that for me now, every day. He has become one of my recent real-life heroes, and there is not a cape, mask or pair of tights in sight. Or maybe there is, but he keeps that side of his life a secret.

Tony recently told me that Milla couldn't speak. She communicated everything with her eyes, her smile and her laugh. However, she could say, 'Mum, yeah' and 'Wuv you'. He told me his enduring memory was from one evening when he was sitting with Milla in his family living room. He asked Milla if she was okay. Milla looked back at him and said, 'Dad, yeah, okay.' It was the only time she had ever said 'Dad'. Tony was speechless and in tears. He told me he doesn't know where she got the strength to say it, but she did, and for Tony, that became his Everest. He could go no higher than that feeling.

Sometimes, it absolutely is the little things in life that make all the difference. Tony scaled Everest that day and didn't even need to leave his living room.

When I told Tony I wanted to include one of his poems in this book, he graciously accepted and then instantly mentioned me in a tweet. 'A special thank you to my friend Ellis, who reached out to me this year, and whose advice guided me through a very tough dark period of depression. A special man and someone I respect for all he does.'

Ironically, Tony doesn't realise how much he helped me during my own battles with mental health. For that, he will always be a hero to me, and I will always be thankful for having such a wonderful friend in my life.

Rob.

Another inspiring character in my life is a young friend of mine by the name of Rob 'Zed' Metcalfe. You may recognise Rob's name from the front of this book, as he wrote and supplied the book's opening foreword. I asked Rob if he would write it after a moment of clarity. The publishers of this book had asked me to start thinking of who I could approach to write either the foreword or a cover quote. To be honest, I had absolutely no idea. I wasn't friends with anyone famous who I could call upon, and there was no one in particular who I felt could add a level of weighted merit to my book. No one, that was, apart from Rob.

Traditionally, getting a celebrity to write a foreword is supposed to give the book a seal of approval. If the Queen of England says, 'This book is good,' then it must be. If it's good enough for Lizzie, it's good enough for me.

I managed to get Brian Blessed to write the foreword for my Everest book, but that only came about after constantly pestering his manager after they had shown me a lot of support in the run-up to both my attempts on the mountain. I think, in the end, they got that sick of me asking that they must have thought, 'Just send him the one you did for Alan'. Because that's basically what happened. Brian hadn't read the manuscript, and nor did I expect him to. So, what his manager sent me was basically just a rehashed version of the foreword Brian had written for Alan Hinkes' book. But because it was so brilliant, having been written for Alan, a true mountaineer, I was over the moon to have the words associated with myself and my little tome of disaster on the world's highest peak. If you read the forewords from the books, both mine and Alan's, you will spot a remarkably similar sounding foreword, almost identical in parts.

The problem in asking a famous person to write your foreword is that the person you are asking is probably far too busy or not interested enough to read what you or your story is about in the first place. It's a token false economy. I didn't want to attach a famous name to this book in the hope that it would ultimately just add a few more sales. Be that as it may, I thought I had best ask a couple of people beforehand just in case, as it seemed to be the thing to do.

The first person I asked was Mark Manson, an American self-help author and blogger, whose book *The Subtle Art of Not Giving a Fuck* I had recently read and listened to on Audible. The book had been a New York Times bestseller and had sold millions of copies around the world. It was perhaps a bit audacious of me to ask, but I have always lived by the mantra of 'Shy bairns get no sweets.' In other words, you don't ask, you don't get. I followed Mark on Twitter, and as luck would have it, I noticed he had put up a tweet in which he said, 'For the next two hours, ask me anything.' Bingo!

'Hey Mark, I have a new book due out, and I was wondering if you would write a quote for the cover, or better still, would you read it and write the foreword?' I confidently tweeted, not expecting a response, if I'm honest. However, I was pleasantly surprised to receive a response less than thirty minutes later, even if I was rejected out of hand.

'No, sorry, but well done on having big enough balls to ask,' he tweeted back.

I guess you can always look to take the positives away from any situation, even in rejection. Always have big enough balls to not be afraid to ask. If you haven't, then grow a pair. A few weeks later, I asked again after he reposted the same tweet, again asking for people to ask him anything. He said 'no' again, but this time wished me all the best with it.

The second and last person in the public eye that I asked was the English writer, broadcaster, former castaway, adventurer, recent Everest summiteer and all-round posh nice guy Ben Fogle. Well, it was his agent I asked, but I knew it would get back to him. I had always admired Ben, ever seen seeing him on that Castaway show on the BBC over 20 years earlier. Marooned on a cold and windswept Scottish island, Fogle was part of a larger group of people who had to come together and fend for themselves for a whole year, living off the island habitat. Ben had since gone on to launch a very successful career for himself in the public eye, mainly as a presenter on British TV of wilderness shows and, rather randomly, the dog show *Crufts*. However, he had shown he was worthy of being asked to write my foreword by rowing across the Atlantic Ocean, racing to the South Pole, running across a Moroccan desert and, in 2017, climbing Everest.

He was heavily criticised after he climbed the mountain as part of team Kenton Cool. Initially, the Olympic Gold Medal-winning cyclist Victoria Pendleton was also part of the team, but she had left to go home early into the climb after failing to acclimatise. I always felt the criticism was harsh. Yes, he had climbed as part of a commercial team, just as I had, and yes, it hadn't cost him a penny to attempt the peak, as he had all his costs paid for by a Jordanian princess, just as I had—no, wait. Apologies, wrong book. That's my novel, coming next year.

The fact is, he still had to put one foot in front of the other and climb the mountain. And as I have always said, I have nothing but the utmost respect for anyone who has climbed the mountain.

His agent responded a few days after I had sent an email asking, with a 'Thank you for thinking of Ben, but sadly it is a no thank you.' She did go on to say that this was because Ben was being inundated at the time, after recently releasing a new book about his life in the wilderness.

Wondering if both Mark Manson and now Ben Fogle realised just how big a mistake they had made in turning down the rights to add their name to this book, the door was now open for me to ask my friend Rob. Rob was never my third choice. He was always the person I had in the back of my mind to approach. And I was delighted when he said he would be honoured.

I had first become aware of Rob a few years previously when a mutual friend of ours began sharing his story on social media. Kate Smith was an old retired ex-schoolteacher friend of mine who had followed my attempts on Everest. She would always comment on my posts and trip updates. At the time, she was my biggest—and possibly the only—fan I have ever had.

Kate began to tell me of her son Rick's partner Jenny. Jenny had a son called Rob, who was battling against a recent cancer diagnosis. Rob was 29, with a wife and young son called Caleb. They lived not far from Keighley, north of Leeds, in a beautiful part of England.

At the time, I was beginning to investigate the possibility of offering treks to Everest through my Everest Dream community that I had built up on Facebook. Kate went on to add how Rob had always wanted to see Everest and that he was still planning to do so. He had no aims of climbing the mountain, but trekking to base camp was a big goal, and he didn't see any reason why he couldn't achieve it. I agreed with Kate.

Jenny, Rob's mum, got in touch with me in January 2019 after ordering some merchandise from the Everest Dream store. I had sent Rob a message a few weeks prior, saying how I would love to meet him and talk about all things Everest. Jenny thanked me for reaching out to Rob and asked if I could personalise a beanie for him, for when he would eventually trek to Everest. I told her, 'Of course; my pleasure.'

I met Rob for the first time around seven weeks later, after I had arranged to meet him at his mum's cottage in North Yorkshire, not far from Skipton. I had been in this part of the world only three months earlier, after giving a sell-out book talk to a packed church hall in Skipton. When I say 'sell-out' and 'packed', what I mean is that I sold 50 tickets. But that was the room limit, so it was still a packed sell-out. It's all relative, I guess. Skipton Oddfellows Society with 50 guests, or Wembley Stadium with 90,000. Both sell-outs.

I found Rob outside the lane where his mum's cottage was tucked away. It was a beautiful little cottage, in the tranquil and peaceful hamlet of Lothersdale. The sun beat down. It was a beautiful day, so we sat outside in the front garden, with the only sound coming from the nearby sheep bleating away and birds chirping and tweeting loudly. Rob had been living there for the past few weeks while his mum Jenny and Rick, Jenny's partner, had been away for a few weeks' holiday. I could see why. It was peaceful and stunning.

Rob told me all about his cancer journey so far and how he had come to be diagnosed with pleural synovial sarcoma, a very rare cancer of the soft tissue. The previous year, in May, he had been to see his GP, feeling groggy and generally under the weather. His GP sent him for an X-ray, which revealed a lung collapse and an unidentifiable object in his left lung. The following month, Rob had surgery to fix the collapsed lung and was told the object was likely a cyst and that it would eventually disappear on its own.

By August, Rob was feeling no better, with chest pain now a constant. Rob had a further X-ray and a CT scan which revealed the object had now doubled in size. It was now suspected of being a benign tumour. Rob returned to his day job as a climbing wall inspector but began to struggle. The pain began to increase and with it so too did tiredness.

A month later, Rob returned to the hospital, where a biopsy was performed on the lump. The specimen was sent off to a specialist team. In October, Rob was informed he had synovial sarcoma. He quit his job shortly after to start treatment. For the remainder of the year, Rob underwent 25 sessions of radiotherapy, and then at the end of January in 2019, he had major lung surgery to remove the tumour.

I was sitting with Rob four weeks after that surgery at his mum's cottage, where we bonded over Everest, adventure and a love of the outdoors. I connected with Rob instantly, and I think the reason why was that he reminded me of a younger version of myself. Here was a young guy, so full of life, so full of zest and a great passion for outdoor pursuits, yet he had been stopped in his tracks by his diagnosis and course of treatment.

As I left that day to head back across to Teesside, I vowed to myself that I would do all I could to help him. I may not have been able to do anything about the cancer, but at least I could do my best to help with other things. Rob wanted to trek to Everest. I told him I would do my best to help with that. Before leaving, I left Rob a copy of my book and told him I would see him again and to keep thinking positive thoughts. I was sure after meeting him that he could kick this thing. Before cancer, he had been a fit and healthy young man, with a love of climbing and mountain biking. He was still that same person. He had been dealt a pretty rubbish hand, but I was convinced he was young enough to recover.

When I arrived home later that evening, Rob sent me a message to thank me for driving all that way to meet him. He said it was great hearing all about my Everest experiences in person, and that he was 'mega proud' that I had signed a copy of my book. He finished by saying he hoped he could be on one of my Everest treks in a year or so. I very much hoped so too, and I was confident he would be. I did not for one second think that the next time I would speak to him he would drop a bombshell.

We stayed in touch for the next few months, mainly through social media. Rob has always been very upfront about his cancer journey, about which he frequently vlogs and shares photos and life experiences and talks about all his fears and insecurities. It's one of the things I most admire about him. He is not afraid to tell the world how he's feeling, whether that be down-in-the-dumps depressed and feeling scared, or top-of-the-world, feeling elated. Cancer is a cruel disease, and none of us knows exactly how we would react to it if we were diagnosed. I would like to think I could be as brave and as honest as Rob has been.

In March, six weeks after our first meeting, Rob called me. I knew he had attended an important check-up with his oncologist to discuss his treatment plan and to see if the tumour had shrunk at all.

"'Weeks to months at worst, 12 to 18 months at best. That is, if you respond well to the chemotherapy,'" Rob told me his oncologist had informed him. If he lived another two to three years from now, that would be brilliant. Rob once told me that from the moment he was diagnosed with his cancer he would prepare for the worst and hope for the best. Sadly, the worst was said much sooner than anyone had hoped.

I put the phone down and cried. Life sure could be cruel. Again, we stayed in touch, mainly through messages and Rob's many Facebook updates. Even in the aftermath of being given the worst news imaginable, his bravery shone through.

In May, a few friends and work colleagues of Rob's organised a charity Everest climb in aid of Rob and Sarcoma UK, the charity funding research into the type of cancer Rob had. The climb took place at the ROKT, a climbing gym in Brighouse, Yorkshire. The outside of the building housed the ROKTFACE, which at 36m high was the UK's tallest outdoor man-made climbing wall. I attended with my mum, Tamara and both the girls.

The idea for the day was—for everyone who wanted to—to climb up the wall and then donate to the cause. Everyone's metres climbed would go towards the total height of Everest, at 8,848 metres. Eventually, the height would be achieved with everyone's accumulative metres added up. When the total was getting close, Rob would get to climb the last few metres onto Everest's summit. It was a brilliant idea, and one I promised I would not miss.

That same morning of the Everest challenge, I had agreed to give a talk at a local scout group in Hartlepool. The talk was only to be a short 15-minute, inspirational-style speech aimed squarely at motivating the scouts. Even four years after my Everest disasters, I was still being asked to give public talks, and it never failed to amaze me. I had agreed to attend and give the talk for free after Alan, the chief scout and local town businessman, who was the CEO of a successful fishmongers, had personally asked me a few months earlier.

'It would mean the world to the Scouts if you could come along and tell them all about your stories of great peril on Everest,' he'd said. 'Of course, you won't get paid, so don't even ask.'

Er, okay, let me think about it, I recall thinking. But that's not what I said.

'Sure, I'd be delighted to do it. Thanks for asking me.'

I told Alan I wouldn't be able to linger long after the talk, as I needed to help climb Everest in Yorkshire. After explaining all about Rob and the challenge, he understood. After I'd finished the talk and spent around 10 minutes speaking to some of the Scouts and their parents, I made my excuses and left, to drive to Yorkshire. Before I left, Alan pulled me to one side and told me that the talk was brilliant, just what he'd hoped for. He placed an envelope in my hand, which contained £100, and thanked me again.

'If you wish to donate it to your friend, please do so,' he added.

When we arrived at the climbing wall after a two-hour drive, the day and the event were in full swing. I could see people going up and down the wall under a brilliant, clear blue sky. We found Rob in the car park, swooning over his recently acquired new VW Campervan, which he had bought so he could spend some quality time travelling around the UK with his wife Beth and son Caleb. I introduced Rob to Tamara, my mum and then Lara and Isla. They all gave him a long cuddle. Tears began to well up in my eyes again. But I composed myself and said, 'Right, come on then, let's go and climb Everest.'

I jokingly said that perhaps it wasn't such a good idea that I went on the wall. 'Look what's happened the last few times I've been on Everest,' I said. 'I wouldn't want to jinx it, not while it's going so well.'

Rob burst out laughing.

As it turned out, I never did get on the wall, as the event was so popular that a queue had formed of people wanting to climb. Lara and Isla both got to have a go, and their metres climbed were added to the rapidly increasing total. Rob introduced me to all his family who were in attendance, including his older brother Chris. Kate Smith was also there, the lady who had first told me about Rob. I think she was a tad disappointed that the Everest climber did not get to climb on the virtual Everest challenge. I suspected this when she said to me very loudly, 'For goodness' sake, is the guy from Everest not even going to have a go?' I wasn't too bothered. Lara and Isla represented Team Ellis very well.

I placed the £100 I had been given for the scout talk into one of the collection buckets, and I donated 10 copies of my book, which I signed. The books sold within minutes, with all the money going to the day's total. It was a simply wonderful day, and the crowning moment came when Rob got to have his go and scale the final few metres onto Everest's summit. Everyone applauded. The mountain was conquered. There were plenty of tears flowing, too, as everyone embraced and celebrated what was a great day.

A month later, again with my mum and Tamara, I drove for a few hours back to the Yorkshire Dales, to a small town called Grassington, to attend a fundraising dinner organised by Chris, Rob's brother, that was being held in Rob's honour. Rob's mum Jenny had invited us shortly after the Everest challenge. She also asked me if I would say a few words after dinner. I told her I would be honoured. The purpose of the evening was to raise funds for Sarcoma UK, but also for Chris, who was fundraising to take on the challenge of climbing Kilimanjaro, again in aid of Sarcoma UK.

That evening after dinner, and before I gave my speech,

I made a special donation to Rob. I had picked up on the fact that Rob's favourite colour was orange, as it was mine too. Most of my outdoor kit was either orange or had some orange in it. On Everest in 2015, I had worn an orange down jacket that had been given to me by the outdoor clothing manufacturer Berghaus. I wore it the day I was in the icefall when the earthquake hit. During my short speech that night, in which I spoke about what makes a hero, I gave the jacket to Rob and told him that I thought it was heroic how he had been handling his whole diagnosis and journey living with cancer.

What Rob didn't know was that I was also about to donate £800. This had been the total I had raised earlier in the year after I had tentatively announced I was looking to return to that mountain for attempt number three. Those who'd supported me previously were more than happy to do so again. But this time I was falling well short of the target. I didn't think I could do again what I had previously been able to do. Things felt different this time out. I shelved the idea and told all those who had donated what I was planning on doing with the money, which was to donate it to Rob, which I did that night. It wasn't much, but it was all I had, and I wanted Rob to be able to enjoy the time he had with his family, by creating memories in his campervan. This could pay for a weekend in Skegness, at the very least. But knowing Rob, this would more likely be a week driving around the Highlands of Scotland.

Regarding Everest, I did seriously look at a possible return to the mountain, which included going as far as to restart a GoFundMe campaign. Rob had even asked me at one point that, when I returned to Everest, would I take a photo of him with Beth and Caleb and take it to the summit with me? He did add that, even if I only got to Camp One again, that would also be fine. My heart and my head wanted to achieve this for him so badly, but I knew I was never going to be able to raise close to the £40,000 I would need for another attempt. It was a miracle I had been able to do so before, twice. In 2019, I felt that ship had passed.

I cemented my friendship with Rob and his family throughout the remainder of the year, and in the summer, I even designed a special T-shirt featuring some of Rob's most famous hashtags and sayings, such as #fightback #refusetogivein #motivation and perhaps his most famous saying, 'Much Love.' I had noticed that Rob would use this to sign off all his video updates and blog posts. I used the T-shirt printing platform Teespring and sold around 40 T-shirts to Rob's family and friends. And yes, you've guessed it, the T-shirt was orange. I gave all the money raised to Jenny, who then passed it on to Rob.

I just wanted to do my little bit to help in any way I could, so I fell back on the one thing I knew how to do, designing T-shirts, and selling them. We stayed in touch for the remainder of the year, and we would chat often.

Rob continued his battle through into 2020, and as the pandemic hit and lockdown began, he was dealt a body blow when he was advised by the Government to shield at home on his own, due to his health. Rob was extremely high-risk. Contracting the coronavirus could ultimately prove fatal.

Rob's oxygen was his young son Caleb, and the thought of not being able to see his son for three months was going to destroy him. I worried about his mental health, as did all his loved ones and close family. You could see from the ever darker and more reflective video updates he was publishing, through his blog on social media, just how much this was affecting him. In late April, I sent him a message asking how he was doing, as I hadn't seen any posts from him for a while. He responded and told me he had been to see Caleb.

He had endured a torrid time and had suffered a dark few days. Time with his son Caleb outweighed the risk of Rob catching the virus. With his health deteriorating, he made the ultimate sacrifice for the sake of love. If Rob caught COVID, that could have been that. But he was prepared to take the risk to spend precious time with his son. I admired him immensely for it.

One thing I was determined to do with Rob once we were able to, when lockdown was lifted, was to take him for a walk up the hill Roseberry Topping. Rob had read about it in my book and then realised there were a few prints of the hill on the walls of the oncology department at Leeds Hospital.

In August, we finally got that chance. Rob drove across in his campervan, and I met him in the car park of the pub at the bottom. My friend Tom came along for the day to capture some photos. We moved slowly and at Rob's pace, and eventually we made it to the roof of Teesside. The views from the top are always spectacular, even more so on a clear day. This was one such day. It was great to see him again, and especially to see him thriving and walking up a hill under his own steam. Rob was told he had 12-18 months at the most left to live. That was 18 months ago. After the walk, we ate lunch in the King's Head, the pub where we had parked. I gave him a copy of Alan Hinkes' book and showed him the page that spoke about the hill we had both just been up.

'See that,' I said. 'Hinkes has done it all: Everest, K2, Annapurna, and this little old hill we have just come down from is his favourite.'

Rob laughed. 'And rightly so,' he said. 'A very worthy challenge indeed.'

A few months later, I was amazed and gobsmacked to see that Rob had been to the top of Ben Nevis with his brother

Chris. I was very happy for him. When all the experts had told him he should be declining, he was doing the exact opposite and gaining strength each day.

I sent him a message to say how proud of him I was. 'You can do anything if you put your mind to it.'

He replied to thank me for everything. He said that my messages of support over the past few months had helped massively, and that he had recently watched my speech from the dinner in Grassington a year earlier. He said it was this that put the idea into his head of trying Ben Nevis. He signed off with 'Thank you for all you do for me, Ellis.' Much Love, Rob.

***

As I write the words to this book, I am pleased to say Rob is still very much here, and he defies the experts every day with his strength, courage and appetite to live. He has a willing openness to share his story, which he does every single day. He still has dark days, where you can see all his fear and angst across his face. But he recovers and pulls himself out of it.

Rob is one of my heroes. I hope that if ever I should find myself fighting a similar battle at any point in my life, I am able to do so with the same bravery and fortitude as he has and continues to show against the odds stacked heavily against him.

Earlier this year, Rob gave me one of the greatest honours of my life when he sent me the following message:

'Me and Caleb got a fish tank yesterday. We are picking up the fish this afternoon. They are small freshwater Tetras. I have named them:

Everest, Kili, Mallory, Norgay, Irvine,
Hillary, Bear, Hall, Fisher,
Ellis.

Yes, that's right, you have made it into my fish tank.'

CHAPTER SIX
MY LIFE AFTER EVEREST

'Being lost isn't always about missed
direction, it's a calling. Sometimes you have to lose
yourself to find other parts of who you are.'
Malanda

The first time I saw Everest up close, I stood fixated
and entranced, gazing at its upper slopes in awe and
wonderment. I had spent two weeks hiking every day to
finally be able to stand at the bottom of the mountain.

Visiting the mountain's base camp is now a bucket-
list tick, which a lot of people from all nationalities and
backgrounds aim to achieve. And rightly so; it is a life-
changing experience, played out in a stunning landscape
among an intoxicating culture. I am lucky to have lived the
experience three times; once on a stand-alone trip to visit
the mountain's base camp, and then twice more on my way
to climb the mountain.

Some of the most vivid memories I have from that
first visit to the mountain involve some of the individuals
I would meet along the way. After seeing the mountain
for the first time that day back in the year 2000, I began
making my way back to Lukla, the mountain village where
most tourists, trekkers and climbers catch flights back to
Kathmandu.

After I'd left base camp, my flight from Lukla was not for another five days. Lukla was a two to three-day hike at best. I had some time to see other things and do a bit more exploring. I decided to hike over a high mountain pass called the Cho La. This pass, at 5,400 metres high, connected the Gokyo valley to the west with the Everest valley in the east. It was a serious hike, one not to be underestimated, and under a full blanket of snow, it would become a serious mountaineering proposition. I was up for the challenge. I hiked to Dzongla, a summer yak-herding station village which had one or two lodges and was close to the start of the pass. I planned to stay overnight there before setting out the following morning to begin my ascent up and over the pass into the Gokyo valley.

When I checked into the lodge that evening, there was just myself and one other lone Chinese trekker in the dining room. I turned in that night, excited at the adventure which lay in store. Little did I realise just what that misadventure would be.

I had lain awake most of that first night in the lodge, shivering uncontrollably in my sleeping bag. I knew this wasn't good, and I knew the signs my body was telling me. I had become ill, and fever was beginning to take hold. When the morning light finally filtered through into my frozen room, I noted that it was snowing heavily.

Through the night, while I had drifted in and out of sleep, interrupted by whatever illness was coursing through my body, two to three feet of snow had fallen and was continuing to fall. Outside had become a winter wonderland. I pulled my sleeping bag tight around my neck, knowing I would be going nowhere that day.

I ended up not going anywhere for the next 72 hours. The only time I left my room over the next three days was to use the bathroom, which was an excruciatingly difficult

160

experience. It was also rather unpleasant. Bathrooms in the mountains of Nepal consisted of nothing more than a hole in a wooden-planked floor, beneath which was six feet of the foulest, most disgusting pile of human waste imaginable. The one in this lodge looked like it hadn't been emptied all season.

On the second day of being confined to my room with a fever, sickness, and diarrhoea, I shuffled my way outside and across to where the bathroom was located across the courtyard. The snow was still drifting down lightly. The floor was now a solid sheet of ice, which I found out to my detriment when I slipped over and crashed onto my side, heavily bruising my ribs. I eventually made it to the hole from hell and collapsed inside, propping myself up on the walls, nursing my now swollen side. I don't remember an awful lot after that. I must have drifted off to sleep in-between bouts of the fever ravaging my seriously depleted body. All I know is that when I went into that cubicle of horrors, it was still light, and when I finally re-emerged, it was dark. The only reason I did leave was down to the lodge owner finding me slumped inside. I might still be there to this day if he hadn't.

A slight, kindly old man, who ran the lodge, had been incredibly tentative so far, popping his head into my room to see how I was, bringing me flasks of hot tea and bottles of water. When he went to check on me this time and discovered I wasn't in the room, he went wandering and found me comatose, with my face a foot away from the pile of unspeakable filth protruding out of the hole.

After he'd helped me back to my room, we deduced that, between the last time he had checked in on me and the time he found me, 10 hours had passed. That meant I could have been in that stinking germ-infested cesspit for several hours.

For three whole days and nights as I lay drifting in

161

and out of a restless sleep, that lodge owner became my Florence Nightingale, constantly checking in on me to make sure I was okay. Three days earlier I'd been a perfect stranger, who only decided to stay at his lodge because it was the first one I reached. He went above and beyond the call of duty and would go on to treat me—a random stranger—as if I were his own son. His compassion and kindness moved me greatly. I eventually felt better and was able to continue down, although weak and a lot slimmer.

My first visit to Everest was tainted somewhat by this incident. It was so bloody typical of me to become ill on my last few days of the adventure.

Of all the places I have been in this world, it is the countries of Southeast Asia where I continually get struck down with illness. I have been to Nepal four times, and I have become ill four times, once on each visit. I have been ill in Tibet, Thailand and China and suffered a terrible bout of food poisoning in Hong Kong.

Shortly after I graduated from university, Tamara and I spent three weeks in Hong Kong, visiting her sister and brother-in-law, who both worked on Hong Kong Island. I was conscious of falling ill, as I usually do in this part of the world, so I had been exceptionally careful, always washing my hands thoroughly and drinking plenty of water.

During the last week, we dined at an English-themed pub. I ordered sausage, mashed potato and peas. After two weeks of eating a rich Chinese diet, it was nice to have something plain and simple. I assumed there was not much chance of catching food poisoning from an English pub.

Wrong!

I spent the next two days in bed in Tamara's sister's apartment, vomiting, with the most horrific stomach cramps.

However, these attacks of the Delhi belly would not deter

me, as they are part of the traveller's experience. To climb the highest mountain in the world, I would need to return to Asia again, more specifically Nepal.

In 2014 and, unexpectedly, again in 2015, I did that very thing in my attempt to climb to Mount Everest's summit. In doing so, I would be achieving a goal I had dreamed about my entire life.

During both years, I aimed to achieve the dream by climbing the same route that Edmund Hillary and Sherpa Tensing had first climbed back in 1953. The route is now largely ascended hundreds of times a year by hundreds of people. I will not say climbers, because not everyone who climbs the mountain is what you would call a 'traditional climber.' Everest is now seen as the ultimate tick on a person's adventure tick list. I was not the classic stereotypical climber, either. I had done my time more than most to earn my shot on the mountain, but I certainly was not the most qualified or experienced individual to be found on its slopes.

Things did not exactly go according to plan.

During the first attempt in 2014, a large ice-collapse occurred, low down on the mountain, early in the season, killing 16 Nepali mountain workers who were carrying equipment up to the higher camps. This, alongside a politically motivated stance by a certain group of Sherpas, systematically closed the mountain for all climbing. In an unprecedented event, this shutdown had large financial repercussions for hundreds of climbers who had arrived on the mountain with high hopes of achieving their life dreams. Not to mention the impact this had on hundreds of Nepalese mountain workers, who relied on the income provided by these guided ascents of the mountain.

Nepal would honour the climbing permits it had issued that year, for one more attempt. Climbers had five years to return and make that attempt. I decided to hop straight back on the plane and return a year later.

I am making this sound very matter-of-fact, but the reality was as far removed from plain sailing as it is possible to be.

Going to Everest two years running was tough, mentally, physically and emotionally. But where it exacted its toll the most was by hitting you in the wallet. You need deep pockets to make an attempt on the highest mountain in the world. My two attempts were no exception. I was not rich. I was not blessed with an abundance of cash to gallivant around the world, frivolously bestowing it on whatever took my fancy.

Climbing Everest was a pipe dream for me. I had failed to reach the mountain several times over before I finally went in 2014. Every time, I was defeated by the finances required, which I found to be insurmountable.

Making it to the mountain in the first place was the real miracle of my life. To return a year later was, quite frankly, a ridiculous notion. But I did.

To discover how I managed to do it, you'll have to read the book I wrote. But here is a little spoiler: it involved designing and selling T-shirts, a bit of ingenuity and a lot of hard work. Whenever anyone reads my story, with ambitions of climbing the mountain themselves, the number one question I get asked is 'How did you really raise the expedition costs?' It really did involve T-shirts. I wasn't lying.

***

In 2015, Nepal was struck by a large earthquake. Thousands of people lost their lives. In the mountainous rural regions of Nepal, as well as in the Kathmandu valley, thousands more were displaced from their homes, which had crumbled and fallen apart during the one-minute-long quake.

164

Aftershocks continued to rumble for several months. The main quake hit during the peak of the country's trekking and climbing season. On Everest, hundreds of climbers had begun moving up to the higher camps, in preparation for making summit attempts later in the season, myself included.

After the earthquake had subsided, I became stranded at Camp One, along with around 170 other climbers from various teams and nationalities. Two days later, I was flown off the mountain by helicopter. I incorrectly stated in my book that 22 people lost their lives that day down at Base Camp when an avalanche of snow, rubble, rocks and anything that wasn't tied down ripped through the heart of the tented community. It is now more accurately recorded that this figure was 19.

Regardless of the number, it is a heart-breaking and devastating amount of people to have died in one incident. I survived by the narrowest of margins, simply because of where I was when the earthquake struck. Had I been down at Base Camp that day, there is a strong possibility I may not have been so lucky. Our camp was flattened. We had lost everything. I was very lucky to leave Everest in 2015 with my life intact.

It is these events, from two years of attempts on the mountain, that formed the basis of the book. But before I would begin to sit down and write that book, I had to come to terms with what had happened on the mountain, and I was having a very difficult time with that. Within a few months of returning home from Everest, I wrote an article for a guest outdoor blog on the events that had occurred. The whole piece I wrote was riddled with notions of failure and disappointment.

These are the opening few paragraphs to that article:

'When I returned home from my failed attempt on Mount Everest this past spring, for the second year in succession, the world, or more to the point, my world was once again turned upside down. A 20-year dream in my life had been in vain. It appears Everest and my ambition to climb it had been nothing but one huge mistake. I fail to take any positives away from the whole sordid affair. My contempt for the mountain has grown stronger daily. I rued the day I saw a photo of the mountain for the first time and thought to myself, "I am going to climb that one day."'

But why was I feeling such strong feelings of regret? It was never a foregone conclusion that I would have triumphed and stood on the summit of the mountain. Just what was I hoping would happen in my life, if I returned from Nepal, successful in my endeavours? Was life suddenly going to explode into a cacophony of colour and happiness? Was reaching the summit of Everest going to make my life complete? Would I reach a Zen-like state of nirvana? Like a monk who attained complete release from desire and suffering? No, no and no. Of course not.

If I could have taken some more time to reflect before writing that scathing article that day, it would have had a completely different more upbeat and positive tone.

What I should have written was something like this:

'When I returned home from my adventure on Mount Everest this past spring, for the second year in succession, I spent the first few months on cloud nine, grateful to have emerged from such an experience completely unscathed. I had shown that, with hard work, anything was possible. I did not get to step on the mountain's summit, but that was only a small part of the overall adventure. I had spent two glorious trips trekking through Nepal's stunning scenery on my way to the mountain and created some lifetime memories in the process. I am so glad that I got to live out this passion. The events will stay with me for the rest of my days. I regret not being able to stand on top of Everest, but I do not regret one thing about going to Everest. I was excited at what now lay in store for me. What new opportunities and adventures would I now experience because of Everest?'

Now let me ask you, which way of describing my two years on Everest do you think is from a healthier, more open mind? Unfortunately, my mind leaned towards the former, more negative summary of events. I suddenly felt directionless. I was not sure what to do with my life anymore. Without Everest, I felt lost and rudderless. I no longer knew who I was. I had lost every ounce of my identity. Would I have felt this way had I returned from the mountain having stood on the summit? Perhaps, perhaps not. It's difficult to quantify. I will never know, unless I go back and finally stand on the summit.

The book I wrote was called *It's Not About the Summit.* If it wasn't about reaching the summit, why did my life suddenly feel like it was?

This way of thinking would begin to invade every aspect of my life, as I would go on to discover, alarmingly and to my detriment. I was struggling to adjust to life without my dream to climb Everest guiding it.

I felt like Clark Kent, stripped of his powers. Clark Kent without powers is no longer Superman. I was no longer Ellis who wants to climb Everest. I was Ellis who tried to climb Everest, and it didn't work out.

To place things into a little more context, allow me to tell you a little story, involving another Clarke. My story would become eerily similar. But I was a few years away from it reaching crisis point, whereas, for this Clarke, his crisis point came sooner.

Clarke Carlisle was a former professional football player, and he had become desperate. He had lost his place in life. He felt he no longer had an identity, a sense of belonging. There was a huge hole in his life that nothing he did seemed to fill.

One cold December day in 2014, Carlisle had reached the end of the road. He reasoned in his mind with what he was about to do. He was not escaping from his problems. It was the answer to them. He felt this would make everyone happy. To Carlisle, it made perfect sense. It would end his misery once and for all. He took two steps onto the A64, a busy dual carriageway in Leeds, and threw himself into the path of an oncoming lorry. Speaking afterwards about the incident, Carlisle said he remembered the impact that day. 'A loud bang, followed by nothing, then lights out.'

In attempting to end his life, Carlisle hoped to end the pain and suffering he had felt since retiring as a professional footballer the previous May. Having spent several years playing for several professional teams, this former chairman of the Professional Footballers' Association looked to have a good future ahead of himself, away from playing the game. However, leaving behind the playing side of the game exacted a huge toll on him, so much so that he convinced himself he had nothing left to live for. Luckily, Carlisle survived the impact and was able to make a full recovery from the injuries he'd sustained as a result. The lacerations, internal bleeding, a broken rib and shattered left knee would heal. But the mental health scars would take much longer to repair.

Carlisle squarely blamed his depression and difficulties coping on leaving behind the sport he loved in the aftermath of retirement. Not everyone seeks the same way out that Carlisle did, but sometimes we do. It is a very real problem, with far-reaching consequences for future happiness for both the sufferer and the sufferer's loved ones.

This loss of purpose, existential angst, call it what you will, does not just affect professional sportsmen and women. It is an adjustment disorder that can roll over into many areas of life. It is usually precipitated by a feeling of a loss of purpose. Without the thing that made the person who they are, self-esteem is shot to pieces. Without Everest as a goal, and without fully realising what was happening to me, like Carlisle, I had also lost my way in life.

The disorder caused me to doubt myself, to hate myself, and to not want to go on living. For four years after returning from the mountain, I lived my life in a state of denial. I would not admit that the problems I was experiencing had been caused by the events on Everest and the loss of the dream.

I have subsequently learned to deal with it much better, but that only came about after things took a dramatic nosedive. I finally fell off the edge of the cliff I had been teetering on, which thankfully for myself and everyone concerned resulted in swift crisis intervention. This mediation ultimately helped me to come to terms with the loss of purpose and self-worth that I had been feeling for several years but doing absolutely nothing about. I had been doing the classic man thing of bottling everything up, continually telling myself I would snap out of it. But I never did, and that was why things took a nasty jolt towards an almost tragic outcome.

I now know that it is always better to see the positives in any given situation and remain optimistic, rather than being bitter and resentful. These negative feelings are, fortunately, now in my past. I came out the other side a much better person for the experience.

'Let us rise up and be thankful, for if we didn't learn a lot today, at least we learned a little, and if we didn't learn a little, at least we didn't get sick, and if we did get sick, at least we didn't die; so let us all be thankful.' – Buddha. I love that. It gets to the essence of harnessing a positive mindset. I am not going to become all motivational and preachy. I will leave that to the Ant Middletons of the world. Ant, a former special forces soldier and now prime time TV star, and people like him, are far better suited for that role than I am. But what these guys say is all true; once you replace negative thoughts with positive ones, you will start to see positive results. It isn't rocket science. It is simple maths, 101. Put negative in, get negative out. Put positive in, get positive out. And that's it. The true meaning of life.

Speaking of which, in this life, things can always be worse, and things can always be better. It doesn't mean you should beat yourself up if things are bad. Note to self: Listen to your own advice from now on.

Let me give you a real-life but made-up example of how a positive mindset trumps the negative. Imagine you lost out to a colleague at work for a promotion, which you felt you deserved because of all the extra overtime you'd been putting in. Your work colleague who has been given the promotion put zero overtime hours in. Let us call this work colleague Dillon.

You later discover that Dillon has been having an affair with your female boss for weeks on end in the run-up to the promotion. Dillon slept his way to your promotion. Dillon is an arsehole. You are not. You have integrity. Karma eventually comes around, and Dillon gets beaten up by the boss's husband when leaving the office one day. He spends two months in hospital, healing from his beat-down. The boss asks you to step into his role. You tell her to go and get fucked, and you hand in your notice, because while Dillon was making out with her, you had used that time wisely, and found yourself a new job with a rival company on better pay, doing the job you had been denied. You win. The beauty of a positive mindset.

I wish I could say that when I returned from Everest my positive mindset kicked in immediately and life went on the up and up. But sadly, you now know that didn't happen. I became Dillon. I didn't sleep with anyone's wife, but I made bad choices. Choices which ultimately led me to be miserable and unfulfilled. And just like Dillon, I became beaten up.

Suffering the effects of the same adjustment disorder that very nearly cost Clarke Carlisle his life, it would take me months and even years for the mental scars to heal. Negativity and animosity coursed through my veins like a bad hit on the devil's heroin. I questioned my motives and whether I had just wasted over two decades of my life on an egotistical game of chance, where the outcome was always uncertain. Why did I go to Everest in the first place? What was I looking to achieve? These were questions to which I had no answers.

Because I was wallowing in self-pity, I felt sorry for myself and expected others around me to feel sorry for me too. It was overpowering. My whole sense of identity and purpose had been a charade, I would continually tell myself. Without the ambition of returning to the mountain for a third attempt, I was empty and miserable. My entire life had been stripped away.

Even just writing that last sentence makes me realise what a downbeat loser I had become.

I had to do some serious soul-searching to claw my way out of the negative dark hole I had found myself lost in. But I kept clawing and scratching and, eventually, with the help I desperately needed, I began to climb my way back up.

I started to replace my negative thinking with a more positive and opportunistic way of looking at my trips to Everest. This positivity had been there all the time. I just needed to ease up on myself and allow the positive aspects of my Everest experience to come to the fore. It would not be easy but, slowly and surely, I was able to allow the positive in and kick the negative out of my life. Once I did, my life after Everest became exponentially a better and more fulfilling place, and opportunities began to come my way. I battled through the negative and was able to fall in love with the mountain all over again. Seeing the two years on Everest for what they were, mind-blowing adventures of a lifetime—okay, misadventures of a lifetime—enabled me to get back into a happy place.

I had survived the two tragic years on the mountain, and I was back with my family. Others had not been so lucky. It was all about perspectives.

My perspective was out of whack with the reality of the situation. I now had a much richer, more fulfilling life than the one I'd had when I left for the mountain. The experiences on the mountain could benefit my life rather than hinder it. From that moment on, I threw myself headfirst into every opportunity that came my way because of Everest, whether that was a speaking opportunity, a podcast interview or some other public appearance. If I were invited, I would generally attend if I were able to. And the invites came thick and fast.

I did radio interviews, TV interviews, website blog interviews; the list went on and on. At one stage, I felt more famous for not climbing Everest than those who had climbed the mountain.

The first few years of life after Everest passed by quickly. I kept myself busy for the first 16 months writing the book.

At the time, this became very cathartic and helped me to deal with the feelings I was struggling to process around adjusting to this life without the mountain.

I didn't know if I would get the book in print, but I didn't let that worry me. I am usually the type of person who rushes headfirst into something, without planning. I believe what will be, will be. If the universe wants the world to read my book, then by hook or crook it will happen.

When the book was finally released, a friend of mine, Andrew, helped me to organise a launch evening at the National Royal Navy Museum in my hometown of Hartlepool. I had invited the British mountaineer Alan Hinkes to attend, and he said he would try his best to make it across. He was in the neighbouring county of Cumbria on the night of the book party, somewhere in the Lake District. Later in the day, he sent his apologies and said he wouldn't be able to make it. He blamed it on the appalling weather in the Lakes that day.

'It's a total pea-souper out there, young lad,' he said to me on the phone in his broad Yorkshire accent. 'And it's chucking it down.' He added, 'Tutt' roads are like rivers.'

Nonetheless, he wished me all the best and said he hoped I had a great night and book launch.

**

As I previously stated I share something unique with Alan. We both have books with a foreword written by Brian Blessed: his *8000m: Climbing the World's Highest Mountains: All 14 Summits* coffee-table spectacular and my catastrophic account of trying to get up one of them. Yep, the great Mr Blessed endorsed both, equally as complimentary, too. Another strange little coincidence we share is that we both have a love and an affection for a little old hill in North Yorkshire called Roseberry Topping. For both my Everest attempts, I trained on and around it, which I mentioned in my book. Alan dedicated a whole page to it in his book. It looks much more impressive nestled in among his heroic tales of climbing K2 and Everest, among others.

The run-in to the book's release had been a complete disaster. Stress levels had been through the roof for weeks. Self-publishing a book, as I would discover, is far from easy. Because I was not being published in the traditional sense of the word, it meant I needed to adapt and to wear many different hats. Being a celebrity or a household name is so much easier. Yes, I know they still must write the book, but they can then send the completed manuscript to their publisher or agent, who then works their magic on it to bring it to life. I had to bring mine to life all by myself. It is a much tougher proposition writing a book when no one knows who you are. And being a no-one means you must work for it. And boy, did I have to work for it.

I want to introduce you to the steps I needed to work through before I could release the book and physically hold a copy of it in my hand. It isn't exhaustive. I could have added a lot more of the issues I encountered, but you will get the idea.

1. Write the book. For most people, this is anywhere from six to nine months. It took me 18.

2. Bin the book and start again because it's rubbish.

3. Repeat steps 1 and 2, three more times.

4. Find a proofreader to look over it. (I was fortunate enough to find an old friend and former dragon boat team member called Emma, who was happy to do this for me.) I also used my Auntie Jean as a backup.

5. Edit the book to make the writing shine or find an editor. (I opted for the latter.)

6. Find the money to pay for an editor. (I opted for a crowdfunding campaign to achieve this.)

7. Make the changes to the manuscript that the editor has

suggested. This involves deleting half of the book again, taking out what you thought were some of the book's best bits.

8. Sulk over the above for a month.

9. Come up with a title for your endeavours.

10. Write the other half of the book, again. Repeat steps 2, 3 and 4 on this new half of the book.

11. Find a cover designer or design the cover yourself. (On this occasion I opted for the latter, utilising my self-taught graphic design skills.)

12. Begin to market the book to your friends and family and anyone else you think might be interested, including Aunt Doris and her neighbour Janice.

13. Launch a presale campaign to see if anyone is even interested in the damn thing.

14. Order a few samples from the printers to quality-check.

15. When the samples arrive, tear your hair out when you spot a gazillion errors.

16. Lose the will to live and threaten to cancel the whole thing.

17. Repeat point 8.

18. Finally, receive a corrected version back from the printers. Sing Hallelujah!

19. Order an initial print run of books and hope to sell them. Luckily, the presale campaign came through for me. I ordered 300 books.

20. Organise a book launch evening with which to hopefully sell 300 books.

21. Receive the books, literally the day of the book launch even though they had been promised a week before.

22. Realise none of the pages marry up in the index. But it's too late, as you now have 300 books with a fucking useless, redundant index.

23. Fuck it.

You see, it's far from easy self-publishing a book. Do not ever let anyone tell you otherwise.

The evening itself was a roaring success. I sold all 300 of the defective books, which included honouring the presale orders. My friend Michael wandered over to me at one point during the evening to offer me his congratulations. He also knew I had mentioned our friendship in the book.

'Er Ellis, I can't seem to find the bits about me in the book. I found my name in the index, but it said I was on page 190. But page 190 talks about you sipping lemon tea in a tea house—'

'Yes, I know,' I shouted back. 'Just please don't bloody ask.'

Apart from the book, the only other thing that went wrong that night happened early on. One of my financial sponsors for the actual Everest expedition in 2015 was a brewery from Hartlepool called Cameron's. I had kept a table back for the brewery's managing director and his family after he had purchased several tickets. The brewery had even supplied a special limited-edition beer for the night, which we christened Everest Ale. We had matched up every ticket sold to every chair available, to make sure everyone had a seat.

But something along the way went wrong. By 8pm, the room at the museum was packed. The brewery MD and his family had not arrived, yet the table I had allocated for them had people sitting around it. Luckily, they were some of my family members and friends, so I told them to shift in as polite a way as I could. They moved without quibbling and sat on stools around the bar. I still don't know what went wrong. As the venue was part of a marina complex, I think a boat pulled up outside in the dock, and several stowaways emerged and decided to gatecrash. That's my theory, and I'm sticking to it.

As the author, and as was customary at a book launch, I gave a speech, using imagery from my expeditions which I had included in the book. I generated a large laugh when I mentioned how the brewery had told me under no circumstances was I to be seen promoting them and their involvement by using anyone under the age of 18. The first photo I sent back from 2015 was a picture of three small Nepalese kids holding my Cameron's Brewery flag. Oh, how we all laughed.

Beer flowed all night long, including the Everest Ale, Live music played, and a special movie was shown which Andrew had produced. The room fell to complete silence while it was shown. It was a very poignant moment of the evening. We even served dal bhat, the classic staple dish of Nepal, as the evening refreshment. At the end of the night, I spent half an hour signing and selling all the books.

I had decided to donate proceeds from the night to Community Action Nepal, a charity I was particularly fond of. This included ticket sales, money from the sales of the book and the beer. We also ran a sealed-bid auction for some signed prints of Everest, which the founder of the charity and first Brit to summit Everest, Doug Scott, had supplied. All in all, the night raised around £3,000 for the charity.

My friend Andrew Drummond had done me proud. It was a gloriously successful night and a great start for the life of my new Everest book.

The following day, this was slightly soured when I received the first review for the book. And it was for one star. And even that, the reviewer said, was because she couldn't leave zero stars. The review was from a lady who hid behind the cloak of anonymity. I had clearly wronged her in a former life.

She had downloaded and read the Kindle version in one

sitting and decided I was a scumbag who'd had no business being on Everest. She said the book, which was appallingly written, looked like it had been done by a 10-year-old, whom, she added, would probably have done a better job. Those were the good comments. There were plenty of others which were not so nice. I remember thinking at least she hadn't spotted the index. You must take the positives when you can.

As someone who is incredibly thin-skinned, the review rankled me. And I would be lying if I were to say it didn't hurt. It did, it hurt big time. However, over the next few days and weeks, five-star review after five-star review followed. That initial scathing review became a distant blot which I began to forget about. As more reviews came in for the book, however, not all of them were so glowing.

I learned to accept that not everyone was going to enjoy the book. Haters will always hate, and you are never going to be able to please everyone. What is that famous saying? 'You can please some of the people some of the time, but you can't please all of the people all of the time.' There was never a truer word spoken—to a book author, at least. I just had to learn to thicken up that skin of mine and toughen my mind to the insults, especially now my head was above the parapet.

It's human nature to recoil from criticism. It stings. No one likes to be the target of criticism's icy tongue. Some of us are better able to deal with it than others. I wasn't aware of just how unprepared I was for critiques, until after I'd released my Everest book. At the time I was being publicly criticised for daring to attempt to climb the mountain, my mental health was already taking a battering. These critical reviews did nothing to help matters.

Just to supply some context to this open and public criticism, I present a list of words used to describe either the book or myself within a few years of the book's release: 'Selfish, pathetic, whiner, needs to grow up, immature, irresponsible, loser, inept, parasite, cretin, disillusioned, ridiculous, unqualified, fish out of the water, a stain on the mountain.' I could go on, as there were plenty more adjectives used to describe me, none of them fit to print in this book. In writing about my two trips to Mount Everest, I was not prepared for the barrage of insults I would experience for doing nothing more than trying to achieve a dream and then writing about it.

I have never understood how someone can take the time out of their day to sit and type mean words at a keyboard, which can then leave their mark in so many negative ways. This always makes me sad. I am possibly sadder for the person who feels the need to do this. The one thing I have learned in this life is that negativity will always rear up in some manner or another. But no matter how negative someone is, I like to think that kindness always wins through.

I am pleased to say that, overall, most of the reviews that have since been left for the book have been positive. But as is the way with human beings, it isn't the positive ones that we tend to remember, no matter how congratulatory and complimentary they may be. The one-star reviews left by Debbie Hotpants and other similar names are the ones that cut deep and tend to mentally scar us. 999 out of 1,000 reviews could all say the book was amazing. One review, however, says the book is rubbish. I will then stew over that one bad review, rather than feel good about all the positive reviews. The brain is a complex and strange thing.

After my experiences on Everest, and with my story now out there, I decided I wanted to keep the mountain in my life one way or another. This, I figured, would help me come to terms with the sense of loss I had been feeling. Whether

I would achieve this by speaking about the mountain to anyone who would listen, or by returning to the mountain for another attempt, I wasn't sure. Even now, seven years after that first attempt, I have kept the mountain simmering away. I never truly expelled it from my system. It's part of who I am. Summit, or no summit. Successful book, or irresponsible loser.

I have since created a community on Facebook for individuals to come together and share their appreciation, love and enthusiasm for the mountain. I wanted this to become a place of kindness and gratitude, a place where negativity is not welcome. And for the most part, that has happened, as over 16,000 group members will testify. I have always tried to use platforms such as Facebook for good. Facebook, and social media in general, when used for the benefit of others, is a phenomenally powerful tool. In the wrong hands, it is a dangerous weapon that can be very destructive. People can be cruel, and we are now living in a time when everyone has a set of tools with which to air their opinion, whether it's asked for or not.

Overall, I think the emergence of social media has been one of the great things that have come about because of the Internet. Without this means of interacting with complete strangers daily, I very much doubt I would have got to travel to places such as Mount Everest in the first place. As with my life after Everest, as it was before, I still maintain an active presence through my social media channels. You just never know what could be around the corner. I don't rule out anything in life, and if the opportunity should once more come knocking, I want to make sure I'm there to answer the front door. By keeping the online Everest community active and engaged, I'm not ready to walk away from that door, just yet at least.

When I look back on these few years of my life after

Everest, I can point to one thing that helped to turn my life around. It was there before I left for the mountain, but it wasn't until I returned home that it became more pivotal in my life. Before Everest, it was something I did casually when the moment presented itself. After Everest, it became a way of life which I excelled at and quite simply fell in love with. And that something was public speaking.

CHAPTER SEVEN
MY ACCIDENTAL SPEAKING DAYS

'There are always three speeches, for every one you
actually give. The one you practised, the one you
gave, and the one you wish you gave.'
Dale Carnegie

I stumbled into public speaking purely by chance. From a
random, out of the blue invitation to speak at a Women's
Institute meeting one day, I would go on to spend five fantastic
years speaking to dozens of organisations and thousands of
people. And I pretty much loved every moment of it.

There were some challenging moments, like the time
during the summer of 2018. I was the guest presenter at my
former secondary school's annual awards evening. I turned
up that night wearing my best waistcoat and tie. It was a
huge honour to be asked back to my old school, especially
to present awards. When I had left the school almost 30
years earlier, most of my teachers and my school reports
said I wouldn't amount to much in life. For that reason,
the evening was very special to me. I had been told there
was a laptop I could plug my slides into, but when I arrived
there was no such laptop. I still needed to give a 20-minute
presentation without my actual presentation. I managed to
get through it by ad-libbing, but it was still a nerve-racking
experience. Note to self: always bring a backup laptop.

From my very first talk in a church hall to 20 retired

ladies to my very last big talk, where I sold out the lecture room at Plas y Brenin, the national mountain training centre in North Wales, there were some incredible moments, and I am so grateful that I got the opportunity to share my adventures all across the UK.

I didn't set out to become a speaker, and I certainly wasn't looking for it. Speaking found me, and from that very first invite to tell my story to the members of the Blackhall Women's Institute in County Durham, I never looked back. I threw myself into every talk with the utmost preparation, showing due diligence to the audience.

For two years before I went to Everest, I was being invited to talk to groups about my dream to climb the mountain. For the next three years after Everest, it was all about the events that had happened on the mountain. I would go on to speak at some very special events and occasions. Sometimes, I would be the headline speaker, telling my mountain tales in front of up to 200 attendees. I spoke about my adventures on the mountain to captivated audiences everywhere, and I was being paid handsomely in the process. To this day, it is still the best-paid work I have ever done. If I'm honest, I would have done it for free.

I also attended a lot of school awards evenings as the guest of honour, where I would present students with their certificates and trophies. I felt like a celebrity, without being famous.

Outwardly, everything looked perfect. Internally, as much as I was revelling in it all, I couldn't help but feel like a bit of a fraud. Feeling like this is a psychological condition in which an individual doubts their skills, talents, or accomplishments. And here I was, being asked to give presentations on my Everest climbs, yet I hadn't reached the top of Everest. This would then kickstart a chain of events within the mind where I would systematically fall apart.

Right, I haven't climbed Everest, and therefore, strictly speaking, I'm not an Everest climber, therefore why are they asking me to speak at their event, therefore why am I even here? I am such a fraud. What was I thinking? God, I'm such a loser! Get me out of here, quick.

It's a strange sensation to be enjoying something while also feeling incredibly guilty for doing so. Welcome to imposter syndrome. This condition can affect the best of us. It's easy to feel like we do not measure up, no matter who we are and how esteemed the circles we move in are.

David Bowie would constantly tell himself he was inadequate. To counteract this, he had an obsessive work ethic, which helped him to manage his low self-esteem. He once said, 'I was driven to get through life as quickly as possible... I thought work was the only thing of value.' Even the multi-talented superstar Lady Gaga once revealed she often feels like a loser kid in high school. She would constantly have to tell herself she was a superstar, just to make it through the day. Tom Hanks admitted, after playing a middle-aged businessman in the 2016 movie *A Hologram for the King*, that he identified with the principal character's lack of self-esteem and self-doubt. 'How did I get here? When are they going to discover that I am, in fact, a fraud and take everything away from me?'

As you can see, this can be very invasive, penetrating all spheres of society. The feeling of being an imposter spares no one, not even Tom Hanks and not even someone like me, a world-famous Everest climber.

Feeling like a fraud or not, I swept it aside as best I could, and for three years after returning home from Everest, I was in demand. I had been registered with several speaking agencies; inspirational speakers, school speakers, motivational speakers and adventure speakers. If there was an agency out there looking for speakers, there was a good chance I would have registered my details. At one point I was making good money from these talks, very good money. An average talk at a school assembly would net me £500 for a talk that would last 20 minutes. That's £1,500 an hour, which isn't bad at all. The problem with it, though, was that it was highly sporadic. I could do a talk one month and then nothing for another two, and then three would all come along at once the following month. I couldn't rely on it to pay the bills, plus I also knew it wouldn't last. It had a limited shelf life, so I decided to just enjoy the ride while it lasted.

Be that as it may, every time I took to a stage or stood up to speak in front of a large audience, I felt amazing. It was like I was getting to live my fifteen minutes of fame over and over.

Throughout my five-year career as a speaker extraordinaire, I entertained with my story of woe and peril on Everest at school assemblies, retired men's groups, accountancy seminars, women's groups, scout troops, brownie troops, boys' brigades, nurses' societies, the Oddfellows society, and I even, rather proudly, managed to keep a room full of octogenarians awake for a full 60 minutes. Even Doris, one of the group's more difficult members, said it was the best talk she'd ever heard. Praise indeed.

I spoke at a Christmas party in a rather fancy venue on the banks of the Thames in London for EDF, a large French/British energy company. The talk itself went very well, but I don't remember much about afterwards, as I hit London with my university pal Steve, who was now working in the city, and Paul Devaney, an Irish climber who had been on Everest both the years I was. We all got blind drunk together till the early hours.

Another memorable keynote I was booked to attend took place in February 2017. The booking came through from one of the agencies I was registered with, which meant that even with the fee I earned for speaking, the agency also made money off the back of me. I was happy with that, as I probably wouldn't have been chosen for the opportunity had it not been for the agency, which had advertised me in the adventure category on their impressive website. I was rubbing shoulders with some pretty impressive speakers from the world of adventure: Ed Stafford, Cathy O'Dowd (first woman to reach the top of Everest from the north and south side) and Debra Searle, who had rowed the Atlantic solo, to name a few. The fact I was chosen at all was quite frankly ludicrous. I was living the dream, alright.

The choice of a speaker is largely negated by budget. Generally, the larger the organisation, the flashier and more highbrow the speaker. I knew my place, and I knew what I could command, which was around the £1,000 mark. I was chosen to give a talk in 2014 at an IT event in Milton Keynes because Bear Grylls had been asked but he priced himself out of it by asking for £100,000. I asked for £1,500 and got the gig. I always regret that. I could have got paid a lot more, but I didn't ask, so I'll never know. But then, I was not Bear Grylls. I was Ellis J Stewart. I was worth a lot more than £100,000 but Bear had priced it down.

I knew there were speakers on the circuit earning 10 times what I was earning, but these were often celebrities or professional sportsmen and women, as well as being Olympic gold medallists. I was nowhere near that category of speaker.

One of the agencies I was registered to accidentally sent me an email once, requesting my attendance at a GSK (GlaxoSmithKline) convention at Lake Geneva in Switzerland. I would be paid £10,000, flown across from London Luton Airport by private jet and put up in the Mandarin Oriental hotel afterwards.

For a fraction of a second, I thought I had finally made it as a speaker. I had hit the big time at last. It was only when I studied the email in more detail that I saw it wasn't intended for me. It was meant for an Olympic gold medal-winning rower. I had been sent the email in error. However, I picked up on the entire email thread backwards and forwards between GSK, the agency and the Olympic rower. The rower wanted £15,000. GSK were only prepared to offer £10,000. The agency was trying to negotiate the price. I thought I would throw my hat into the ring, seeing as how I'd been made aware of the situation.

I said, 'I know this wasn't intended for me, but if he (the greedy Olympic Gold Medallist) isn't willing to budge, I'll do it for £2,000, providing I can fly from Newcastle Airport.'

The agency responded and told me thanks and that they would let me know. Guess what? I didn't get it.

The one I did get in 2017, however, was for an annual conference called Peak Performance, Performance Matters. It was an accountancy event aimed at taxation through challenging times. I was part of the line-up of speakers nestled among taxation specialists and other accountancy experts. I was to provide the motivational light relief during the day's proceedings, shortly before lunch. The event took place at The Belfry Hotel just outside Birmingham. I travelled down the night before, taking full advantage of the hotel's exquisite facilities. That meant I used the gym and had a steak dinner in the restaurant before hitting the sack.

On the day of my talk, the company had provided each one of the 200 delegates in attendance a copy of my book. Before being introduced, the previous presenter, who had just finished lecturing on taxation in the 21st century, wished me good luck. 'If you can get a smile out of this miserable bunch of bastards, you're better than me,' he said.

I quickly searched for an accountancy joke on my phone, and when I took to the stage, I figured I would recite it to break the ice.

'A woman was told she only had six months to live. "Oh my God!" said the woman. "What shall I do?" "Marry an accountant," suggested the doctor. "Why?" asked the woman. "Will that make me live longer?" "No," replied the doctor. "But it'll seem longer."'

It did the trick; the room erupted in sniggers and general moans of laughter. From the very first moment, I had them in the palm of my hand, and I delivered one of the best speeches I had so far given. It was the talk where I felt as though I had finally arrived as a professional speaker. I was not intimidated by the audience, and they gave me a rapturous round of applause at the end. The feedback received from those in attendance at lunchtime let me know I'd done a good job. I was even asked to sign several copies of my book. I drove back up north very content and £1,300 richer, along with a free overnight stay under my belt and a scrumptious evening meal. Life could be very good as a speaker.

It wasn't all about earning money and not giving back. I was more than happy to offer my services for free if it were for a worthy cause—especially if the cause were in any way connected to Nepal, as a talk I would give later that year would be.

Tony McMurray was a friend of mine whom I had got to know in the run-up to my Everest climbs. He was the financial director for a large American IT company based in Milton Keynes. He was out in Nepal, taking part in a trek to the mountain, in 2015 when the earthquake hit. We met up at base camp a day or so before all hell would break loose and shared some breakfast. In the summer of 2017, Tony had selflessly, out of his own money, arranged for and flown his guide Sukman, from his trek in Nepal, to travel over to England and stay for a week at his and his wife's B&B in Towcester. During the week, Tony took him on a whistle-stop tour of the south of England. He also organised a charity night, with all the proceeds raised being given to Sukman. This was to help with the reconstruction costs of his village in the mountains of Nepal after it had been badly damaged during the earthquake.

Tony asked me if I would attend and give a speech, alongside him and Sukman. I couldn't possibly say no. Tony had advertised the night as an evening with cheese and port and 90 minutes of enthralling mountain madness. He sold 100 tickets at £15 each, and they promptly sold out.

That evening, I also donated, sold and signed 30 copies of my book, from which I handed all the proceeds to Sukman. Tony put me up for free at his B&B and covered all my food and drink while I was his guest. It was a magical evening, catching up with some old friends. The last time I had seen both Tony and Sukman was in Lukla, in the mountains of Nepal, shortly after the earthquake. I didn't, for one second, think that if I ever saw both again it would be in The Saracen's Head public house in Northamptonshire, scoffing cheese and glugging wine. Have I mentioned that life moves in mysterious ways yet?

***

Of all the presentations and talks I would go on to give over the few years after Everest, without a doubt the most challenging one I agreed to do took place shortly before my book launch in November 2016. The venue was to be someone's home—well, it was a marquee in a garden in Wiltshire, but it was still in the grounds of someone's home. That someone was a lady by the name of Liz, who was the trustee for a charity called Kidasha. This was a UK-based charity, which provided education, healthcare and the possibility of a better future to vulnerable children in Nepal.

It ended up being particularly tough, as I was poorly throughout the whole event with raging flu. It was a talk I had agreed to do for free, as it was in aid of Nepal. The one thing I'd told myself was that I would never turn down the opportunity to raise money for Nepal's impoverished people, so this was very much a case of 'Suck it up, big boy, and get on with it.' The organiser of the event had sold out the talk weeks ago, and over 150 people would be in attendance at £25 per head. I couldn't let them down. It was also a great opportunity to push my book, which was due for release in a matter of days.

I drove down to Salisbury from my home in the north-east a day earlier, feeling like death warmed up the whole way; a torrid five-hour car journey. When I arrived at the village where the house was, I saw my mug shot everywhere. It was on the village hall noticeboard and stuck to every lamppost I passed. They had certainly done a grand job advertising the evening.

Liz had graciously allowed me to stay over at her house. I spent the whole of the next day shivering uncontrollably in her guest bedroom. I managed to force myself out of bed an hour before I was due to talk, but only just. I drank a whole 300ml bottle of Metatone tonic and somehow managed to hold it all together and give an 80-minute talk on my experiences on Everest. I received a standing ovation at the conclusion and even took over 50 pre-orders for the book. I was desperate to get back to bed upstairs in my host's house, but a 90-year-old chap called Fred, who'd once visited Nepal in the '60s, was keen to converse with me. Forty minutes later, I collapsed back into bed, where I slept for a solid 10 hours, missing a pre-arranged breakfast with Liz and her family the following morning.

Before I set off on the drive back up north, I had

191

planned to stop off and visit Stonehenge, as I'd never been there before. I told Tamara over the phone I was going to do it and then set off after that. I pulled into the car park at Stonehenge and made my way to the visitor centre. Before I could get a ticket, I rushed to the toilets and vomited all over a toilet bowl. I reported the mess to the front desk, who informed me not to worry about it. I left, got in my car and somehow managed to drive the five hours home. When I arrived home, Tamara asked me what I thought of Stonehenge. I replied that I had absolutely no idea.

It wasn't one of my better experiences of public speaking, but I'd got through it, and that was what counted. Plus, it was for a Nepalese-benefiting charity. All in all, I think the evening raised over £5,000. I even donated proceeds from my book sales, so I'd have to say it was worth it, even if I did feel like I was at death's door throughout the whole experience.

***

One of my more memorable public appearances had happened a few months earlier, when I was invited to speak and present awards at a royal palace, in the presence of royalty, no less. In the summer of 2016, a full year after Everest, a very formal-looking letter came through the post. It was an invitation.

'The Equerry-in-Waiting to the Duke of Edinburgh is desired by his Royal Highness to invite Ellis J Stewart to attend and present Awards to Young People who have achieved a Gold Duke of Edinburgh's Award in the Gardens of the Palace of Holyrood House on Monday, 4th July 2016.'

The invitation went on to add that dress for the day should be a lounge suit or Highland dress. I had no idea what a lounge suit or a Highland dress was. I'm allergic to wearing a tie at the best of times, but for this occasion, I would need to spruce myself up to the nines. Of course, I accepted in kind. It's not every day one receives a royal invite! I was incredibly honoured to have been asked. I could take two guests, so that meant Tamara and Mum could attend with me.

When I discovered that 'lounge suit' just meant formal, I had to go out and buy a suit. I had only ever owned one suit before in my life, and that one had the England football badge on the right chest. I just didn't do posh. Casual was my middle name. In fact, if you look up 'casual' in any English dictionary, it'll say something like 'relaxed and unconcerned'. It might go on to add 'See also Ellis J Stewart.' I am a flip-flop and tank top kind of guy, that's for sure.

The day we drove to Edinburgh, I had scrubbed up impeccably. I was unrecognisable. On the way, we stopped off for fish and chips in Berwick-upon-Tweed, where I managed to spill grease down the front of my suit. I scrubbed the worst of it off with a pack of baby wipes in the public toilets in the middle of Berwick town centre.

When we arrived at the palace, we were met by my official chaperone for the day, a lady called Lisa, from Cumbria County Council. I was there that day to present awards to around 30 young people from Cumbria. Before meeting the Duke of Edinburgh himself, I was to give a short inspirational speech to my group, their parents and watching dignitaries. To say I was nervous was an understatement. I had written a speech specially, which honoured the achievements of those receiving their awards and paid tribute to the award itself. As a Duke of Edinburgh Gold Award holder myself, it felt very apt.

I had achieved my award just before turning 25. I was

living in Milton Keynes at the time, but I always like to say Buckinghamshire when I talk about this period of my life, as it sounds way posher. I had just snuck in before I was too old to complete it. Turning 25 was the cut-off. Like everything else in my life, I had started my award in my early twenties, but I hadn't bothered to complete the final few sections. Procrastination is a bitch. One of the remaining sections I had left to complete was the best of the lot: the expedition. An 80km self-sufficient journey on foot in a wilderness environment. This had my name written all over it. Buckinghamshire County Council had put me in touch with several individuals to complete the expedition. Later that summer, I spent four days and three nights hiking around Ben Nevis and Fort William with four early 20-something females. It was a hardship, but someone had to do it.

As I stood on the lawn of the palace that day with hundreds of pairs of eyes all focused on me, I nervously but confidently began to speak. A bead of sweat ran down my temple.

'Ladies and Gentlemen and Award winners, it's an honour and a privilege to be here today to be presenting DofE Gold Awards to all these magnificent young people. As a Gold Award holder myself, I recognise the magnitude of the achievement. But not only that. I also recognise the dedication, hard work and commitment that goes into the achievement of the award.'

With the formal introduction out of the way, I thought I would mix the next part up a bit. I cleared my throat and, gaining more confidence, loudly spoke.

'As a means of an introduction to who I am, I want to read you one of my old school reports,' I began. '"Ellis just simply doesn't try hard enough. He has a couldn't-care-less attitude, which does not do him any good. He is lazy and bone idle, and unless he pulls his socks up, I worry for his future."'

I looked up to see stunned expressions on people's faces. I continued, 'One line from that report stung more than the others. "He doesn't try hard enough." From that moment on, I vowed for the rest of my life that I would try hard enough.'

Everyone smiled. Mission accomplished.

I carried on delivering as polished and as slick a short inspirational speech as I had ever given.

'When I achieved my award, it was one of the proudest moments of my life at that moment in time, just as you should be incredibly proud of yourselves,' I said. 'And I am sure your parents, other family members and friends are just as proud. I do not doubt that achieving my gold award set me on the path of adventure that ultimately enabled me to attempt to climb Mount Everest, twice. I embrace every single day and live every day as if it's my last.'

I knew I was giving a good speech which was said with complete and utter conviction, because I believed in what I was saying. I finished with the following:

'In life, it is far easier to not take the risk and to not take the adventure in the first place. But then life would be boring. A ship in a harbour is safe, but that is not what ships are for. They are meant to sail the oceans and explore. You are all here today celebrating the achievement of your awards because you made that commitment to get up off your sofas and do something with your lives. You are all now Gold Award holders, and every one of you is a hero. It would have been far easier to stay on that couch watching Game of Thrones.'

It was a bit cheesy, but it worked out well, and it got the message across that I was trying to convey, which was, basically, if you want something in life, then work your backsides off until you get it.

After I had the met the Duke of Edinburgh himself, Prince Phillip, and he informed me that my story was better than climbing Everest anyway, I presented his awards and got the formalities out of the way.

I heard a voice in the tented-off area neighbouring ours on the palace lawn. Another group of young people were also receiving their awards from their honorary guest, and I recognised his Yorkshire twang immediately. It was the British mountaineer Alan Hinkes, who was most famous for being the first Brit to climb all 14 of the 8,000-metre peaks. Quite the achievement. Queue an almighty attack of imposter syndrome. I couldn't believe it. Here I was, rubbing shoulders and sharing the stage with mountaineering royalty, as well as actual royalty. I recall thinking What the actual fuck! All I had done in my life was attempted to climb Mount Everest. Twice. And I had come up short both times. In Alan, you had a real climber. The guy had done it all. 'Annapurna, K2, Nanga Parbat, Everest,' you say. 'Been there, done that. Got the T-shirt, mate. And here; while we're at it, hold my pint of Tetley's while I climb up the side of this palace.' He was as worthy an honorary guest as you could find gracing Holyrood palace that day. I had no idea what I was doing there. Damn you, imposter syndrome! Damn you to hell.

The Duke of Edinburgh retired from public duties, not long after the summer of 2016. I think that day in Edinburgh was one of HRH's final public appearances, and I got to be there in attendance and meet him, alongside my wife and mum. It was a special day. But then there were lots of special days in the few years after coming down from the mountain. It is true what I said: the mountain, and my failure to conquer it, had opened doors and possibilities I don't think would have been there had I climbed to the very top.

Just a few days after the Duke of Edinburgh Awards, I found myself in East Yorkshire. This time, I was the guest of honour at Hymers, an independent school in the heart of Hull that was steeped in a 120-year history. Once again, I had been booked through one of the agencies I was represented by: School Speakers.

On this occasion, I was paid to spend all day in the school, delivering workshops to some of the younger students. In the evening, it was time for the annual awards. I was to give a short inspirational speech and then hand out the individual awards and prizes. If you can imagine being asked to give a speech in the great hall at Hogwarts School of Witchcraft and Wizardry, then you wouldn't have been far away from that at Hymers. Standing on the stage that evening, gazing around at the almost-300 parents and students in attendance, the great banquet hall from Harry Potter is exactly what it reminded me of. I half expected a sorting hat to appear at any moment, to place the students into their respective houses.

Through all the formality and tradition that day, I was made to feel incredibly welcome by the headmaster and other staff members, and coming so soon after the awards in Edinburgh, it was another special occasion, one which I remember with fondness.

In late 2018, I decided it was time to bow out of speaking duties. I felt I had done all I could and spoken about Everest and adversity more times than I cared to remember. Talks and opportunities had begun to dry up, and I knew I was reaching the end of the road. I decided I would try to go out on a high. In the autumn, I began to advertise and sell tickets for a mini book tour. It was the one thing I hadn't done at the time the book came out, and now, two years down the line, I decided it was time I did something about it.

I wasn't fortunate enough to have an agent who could organise this on my behalf, so everything fell upon me to sort. I didn't mind; I was generally good at this sort of thing. I began to look at venues in several areas of the country, recoiling in horror at the hiring costs for almost everywhere I considered. I took suggestions from people for places I should look at and would then promptly contact the venue. I was realistic in my endeavours. I knew I wasn't going to fill the Royal Albert Hall, or any large hall, for that matter. I was more interested in the smaller, more intimate venues, the kind that would hold 50 people at the most. I was confident I could put bums on seats if I kept the price reasonably low, so I sold tickets for £10. The three venues I immediately began advertising were Plas y Brenin, a national mountain centre in the heart of Snowdonia National Park in North Wales, the Oddfellows Society in Skipton and a hotel in Penrith in the Lake District. I had taken advice from a book publisher who had advised me to stay away from main towns and cities. They are harder to sell tickets for, I was informed, as you are competing with whatever else may be happening that evening, such as theatre, comedy clubs, cinema, etc.

I heeded that advice and looked for more rural-based locations and venues. The three I had selected were perfect. I couldn't imagine there was an awful lot to do in Capel Curig in Wales on a Friday night in November, and even less in Skipton a few days later, a Sunday night.

Straight away, I was having success with the Welsh venue and Skipton. Tickets were not exactly selling like hotcakes, but they were selling, and that was what counted. However, I hadn't sold a single ticket for the hotel in the Lake District. In organising the venue in Wales, I'd done it all off my own back. With the other two venues, I'd worked with a girl called Mel, who ran an events company called

Due North. I had noticed that she had recently organised a talk for Doug Scott, which had sold out, so I contacted her to see if she could help me. She jumped on board and got to work on Skipton and Penrith, but Penrith remained stubbornly uninterested. With the date of the Penrith talk fast approaching, we decided to pull the plug, having not sold a single ticket.

The venues in Skipton and Wales, however, had both almost sold out. I decided those two venues would have to do. I needed to be realistic, after all. I wasn't a household-name mountaineer. I was just Ellis, the misadventure king from County Durham. I hadn't achieved anything of note in my life, yet somehow I had spent the past few years in the public eye as a sort of after-dinner motivational speaker. I would take what I could get. After selling over 100 tickets for the North Wales event and 50 for Skipton in North Yorkshire, I was happy.

Plas y Brenin in Capel Curig had been at the heart of training outdoor instructors for generations. Built originally as an 18th-century inn, it remained a hotel for over 150 years. In 1955, it was acquired by the central council for physical recreation and turned into a national recreation centre. It has been at the forefront of outdoor education ever since. The area around the centre was also rich in history. It was the mountains and villages around Capel that the 1953 British Everest team had used as a training base, before heading out to the mountain. The whole area had strong ties to Everest. Plas y Brenin was a fitting venue in which to tell my own stories of the mountain.

That night, there was not a spare seat to be had. Over 120 people crammed into the main lecture hall, and more people turned up and paid on the door. I had travelled down to Wales with Andrew Drummond, my friend who had helped with the book launch. He was there at the start, so I figured it would be nice for him to be there at the end. Plus, we had decided to make a weekend of it and stay over in the centre and go off out into the hills of Snowdonia the following day.

I told my story that night in two parts, taking a 30-minute interval in the bar to allow people to stretch their legs and replenish drinks. It was also an opportunity to sell the book. The rule of thumb, I had been told, with a book evening was to expect to sell 10 percent of books to the total number of people in attendance. So, for 120 people, I should sell just 12 books. By the end of the interval, I had sold and signed over 30. At the end of the talk, I sold another 20. I almost sold a book to over half the people in attendance. A lot of people who didn't purchase one came up to me and said they already had a copy, and that was the reason why they were here. They had read the story and now wanted to listen to it live. I felt humbled and incredibly proud of the journey I had been on.

The feedback from the evening was phenomenal, and I felt like I had just lived my finest hour, delivering my finest presentation. Everything worked, and everything came together. For once, the misadventure fairies had decided to give me a wide berth. They must have decided to let me have my night. They would be back; of that, I had no doubt.

Back in my room that night, I found a card and a bottle of wine on the bed. It was from Tamara. She had arranged for the staff from the centre to deliver it. She said how proud of me she was for taking this thing as far I had taken it, and to enjoy every moment of the night. Which I thoroughly had.

The following day, Andrew and I scrambled up the north ridge of Tryfan. The weather was glorious, clear blue skies and crisp winter air. We were even rewarded with a Brocken

Spectre near the summit, a spectacle in which you see your shadow cast onto a nearby cloud opposite the sun's direction. The shadow is accompanied by halo-like coloured rings which make the whole effect an ethereal, almost heavenly, phenomenon. The universe had my back and was letting me know in its own little way.

Once we came down from the hill, we stopped at the Pen-y-Gwryd hotel in the valley, a place of pilgrimage for mountaineers the world over. It was here that members of that 1953 team had stayed when training for Everest. Nowadays, the hotel was a shrine to the team, with artefacts from the expedition on display in the bar area and the team's signatures still visible in ceiling panels. It was one of the best mountaineering hotels in the world, and you couldn't come to these parts and not visit it. We had a pint, paying tribute and silent prayers to those conquering heroes before departing for the long drive back north.

The following day, I would get to do this all over again and tell my story to the fine folk of old Skipton town. The Oddfellows society venue had, like Plas y Brenin, sold out, the only difference being the venue was much smaller, catering to just 50 people. The evening was a lot more personal and cosier, made all the more special by the presence of an elderly lady and her husband who I had often spoken to online but never seen face to face. Kate Smith had been a big fan of mine during both attempts on Everest. It was lovely to finally meet her, and doubly so that she got to sit and listen to my story in real life rather than reading it through the pages of my book. It was Kate who would go on to introduce me to Rob Metcalfe a few months later.

And that was that. I was confident that I had spoken my last word in public. I had told my Everest story to death. It was time to put it to bed. I never imagined, after giving a talk for the very first time to the Blackhall Women's Institute five years earlier, that I would go on to speak over 100 more times, to audiences from all sorts of backgrounds. From Swindon to Edinburgh and lots of places in-between. I had lived and loved mostly every moment of the journey. I would have loved every moment unequivocally if it had not been for that damn imposter syndrome making me feel like a fraud, every time I stood up to speak. I dare say I would possibly have been still speaking to this day. I attended one or two more primary schools as a favour to some friends and inspired tiny minds to never give up on their dreams, and I also gave an after-dinner speech at Rob Metcalfe's charity dinner the following summer. But other than that, I was finished. Douglas Adams, a British author and satirist and writer of a favourite book of mine, *The Hitchhiker's Guide* to the Galaxy, famously said, 'I may not have gone where I intended to go, but I think I have ended up where I intended to be.' I couldn't agree more, and the sentiment perfectly echoed my time as an accidental and motivational public speaker.

***

With new horizons now out there to behold and new opportunities to seize, I looked towards the tide. It was time for the tide to wash those opportunities upon the shore, to my feet. But with every new tide and each new day, those opportunities refused to come in. Eventually, I realised I would have to find those opportunities myself. They were not going to come to me. I would need to be proactive in finding them.

It soon dawned on me that I was facing up to the greatest challenge of my life to date. A new year would soon come around, and so began a tumultuous and testing 12-month period. The misadventure fairies were back, alright. And this time, they were determined to dance on my grave. The biggest battle of my life had just begun.

CHAPTER EIGHT
MY ROOM IN HELL

'You can't stop the waves,
but you can learn to surf.'
Jon Kabat -Zinn

One of the best descriptions of depression I've read is by
a lady called Martha Manning, a psychologist who wrote
a book in the mid-90s about her spiralling descent into a
severe depression. In it, she said this: 'Depression is such a
cruel punishment. There are no fevers, no rashes, no blood
tests to send people scurrying in concern, just the slow
erosion of self, as insidious as cancer. And like cancer, it
is essentially a solitary experience; a room in hell with only
your name on the door.' I was given a ticket to this room
in 2019, and I spent several months within its four walls,
unable or unwilling to escape.

In January, I attended a talk given by a rather colourful
individual. Tom, a good friend of mine, had recently
interviewed a true-crime author by the name of Jamie
Boyle, a former boxer who had swapped his boxing gloves
for the writer's chair and had made a successful career for
himself writing the true-life memoirs of several North-East
criminals. On the evening in question, Jamie was hosting a
live Q&A at a venue in Stokesley, North Yorkshire, with his
most recent book subject, Brian 'The Taxman' Cockerill.
Tom invited me along for the evening to keep him company,

and possibly more so because he was scared to go alone. When we arrived, I couldn't say I blamed him.

In his heyday of the late '80s/early '90s, The Taxman had been one of the most feared men on Teesside. Working as a Mafia-style crime lord, he would visit the region's drug dealers and then charge a levy on their ill-gotten gains. This ultimately led to many violent encounters and street fights in a career that stretched some 30 years.

That night in the bar, a now 54-year-old Brian sat on a stool, wearing a crisp white sports tracksuit. He wouldn't have looked out of place if he had just strode out onto the centre court at Wimbledon, with a bag slung over his shoulder and tennis racket in hand, apart from looking like Reggie Kray on steroids. He was a big strapping fella, and I certainly wouldn't have wanted to have had a meeting with him about any of my tax affairs back in the day.

He spoke confidently and matter-of-factly about his life of crime living on Teesside. His stories of kneecapping drug dealers and beating the living shite out of people certainly added an interesting dynamic to the evening—a bit different to my stories of surviving avalanches and raising money by selling T-shirts. Looking around the bar that night, it was a who's who of some of the region's most infamous ex-criminals, all now reformed characters. I had never felt so nervous in all my life. I didn't think there was much chance of anything kicking off, that was for sure. Nobody would have dared.

One of the things that amazed me most from Brian's talk was the fact that here we had a guy who, for over 30 years, had lived and operated in a seedy underworld, dealing with some proper reprobates and shady characters. Now, he was up speaking, telling his stories of how he'd dished out his retribution, like Jesus preaching to the masses after his resurrection. This self-titled Taxman had recently decided he wanted to help people, to prevent others from, as he put it, 'making the same mistakes I did and treading the same path.'

He once had to have over 170 stitches following a violent attack. 'I lost two pints of blood that night, too,' he casually said.

Brian would spend time behind bars, and it was here that he saw how many young people were in prison. After that, he decided he was going to change his life and try to reach the youth of Teesside. He was also very candid about his battles with mental health and depression.

'I want to deliver a message of "Don't suffer in silence,"' he said. 'There is no shame in admitting you have a problem.'

Brian was now mostly spending his time visiting schools and youth clubs, spreading his anti-crime message. 'I want to let these kids know that a life of crime isn't all that glamorous,' he added. 'It's not bleeding *Lock, Stock and Two Smoking Barrels*.'

I came away that night seriously impressed that an individual such as Brian, who'd been heading for life's scrapheap, had transformed his fortunes and wasn't afraid to admit his failures and faults. He was now doing something positive in the local community, and to me, that was highly commendable. No matter who you are or where you are from, we all have the ability to change. In this case, Brian had decided once and for all to change his felonious ways and life of crime. In doing so, he would become a motivational preacher, spreading his new positivity, anti-crime message to young people across the region.

Feeling incentivised and inspired, I would begin the year with much optimism and hope. It was a new year, and I wanted to make sure it was going to be a good one. It wasn't long before the wheels of motivation would come hurtling off. I was about to become the most demotivated and discouraged I had ever been.

Everything began to unravel at an alarming pace in early March, after I had returned from a trip to Nuremberg in Germany. I was there to attend an international trade show called the IWA Outdoor Classics, the world's leading trade fair for hunting, shooting sports and equipment for outdoor activities. I was to help on the stand of a US brand from Montana called Cold Avenger, which manufactured and sold cold-weather face masks. At the time, I was exploring the possibility of working for the company, either as their guy on the ground in Europe or by relocating across to Montana and becoming involved in all aspects of the company. I was heavily for the latter, and I even began researching house prices and living costs. But sadly, nothing came of it.

I was introduced to John Sullivan, the owner and CEO of Cold Avenger, by his sister Carol, a lady from Orlando in Florida, who I had become very good friends with after she'd read my Everest book. Carol, along with John, had financially supported the campaign I started to bring that book out as a hardcover in 2018. John was a retired professor of emergency medicine who loved skiing and outdoor activities. He developed the Cold Avenger face mask as a way of preventing cold air from getting into the lungs when taking part in outdoor activities. It was particularly helpful in places like Montana, where the outside temperatures in winter could drop off the charts.

Cold Avenger was in Germany, exhibiting at the show to try to make inroads into the European market. Carol had arranged for me to help due to my outdoor background and recent trips to the Himalayas, which John thought would be a good talking point on the stand. I also took with me several copies of my Everest book, which I used to promote the book and drum up sales on Amazon in Germany.

I almost missed the flight to Germany, as the meet-and-greet car park company I'd used to leave my car with didn't meet or greet me. I was left high and dry, with nowhere to leave my car. With only an hour till my flight was due to depart, I swung into the premium parking area at Manchester Airport and agreed to pay a zillion pounds for three days' parking. I'm sure the company who deserted me are in cahoots with the airport. They probably get a kickback from the extortionate fee I had to pay.

I had only been to Germany once before in my life, and that was in the mid-90s as part of the dragon boat team. We took part in an international festival in Stuttgart. I remember it well through the haze of all the alcohol that was consumed. The team travelled everywhere in our coach, and Germany was no exception. We all met in a local pub the night we would drive down to Dover for our ferry crossing into France, and then onto Germany. This was a big mistake. The drinking started at 7.00pm, continued through till 11.00pm and then carried on for another 830 miles and 14 hours. It was a very fragile and heavily hungover team of supreme professional athletes who finally rocked up in Stuttgart, ready to race the cream of Europe's top paddling teams. The words cherry and brandy should not exist in the same sentence, and I will never touch another drop of the stuff for as long as I live.

We would go on to win the event in Stuttgart, but the most memorable part of the weekend was having my name sang back to me by hundreds of people at a beer festival we attended. A British band called Smokie had a huge hit around the world in the 1970s with a song called 'Living Next Door to Alice'. The song had even reached number one in Germany, so it's fair to say it was popular. To make matters worse, the song had recently been given a new lease of life with a new version of the song, featuring Chubby

Brown, a foul-mouthed British comedian. Roy Chubby Brown, who was famous for songs such as 'Dolly Parton's Tits' and 'My Dog's got Tourette's', added his own unique words to the song, which suddenly became 'Alice, Alice, who the fuck is Alice?' Yes, I know it's not saying 'Ellis', but when you hear the song, it sounds exactly like they're singing my name. Every time the chorus came around, everyone—and I mean everyone—belted out at the top of their lungs 'Ellis, Ellis, who the fuck is Ellis?'

Thank you to Smokie and Roy Chubby Brown for ruining the next few years of my life. Whenever I went away with the team, I would have to endure that song being sung back to me at every opportunity.

Back to my most recent trip to Germany. When I'd landed in Nuremberg, I took a shuttle to the old town area of the city and immediately hit a problem. I could not gain access to the apartment I had booked through the accommodation site Booking.com. The access code I had been emailed didn't grant me access. By now I was tired, irritable and hungry. Not a good combination. I called the number I had been given, and through a spattering of German words I understood and some broken English, I was able to discern that a new code would be emailed to me.

I waited for an hour outside in the pouring rain, before giving up and dragging my bags a few blocks to the hotel where the Cold Avenger team were staying. John said that if I were not able to get into my room, I could always crash in one of theirs. Luckily, the problem got resolved later after a new code was sent to me. A hot shower had never felt so good.

All told it was a fabulous short visit to Germany, and it brought back memories of my first visit over 23 years earlier. At the show, I enjoyed immensely chatting with the visitors who came over to our stand. I had to get to grips with the product, so I had a quick crash course in all things Cold Avenger. After that, I was away, chatting to anyone who showed a glimmer of interest. It took me back to the days when I'd been a sales rep for an outdoor clothing brand. I've always been a very good salesman. I could sell underwear to a nudist and religion to the Pope, given half a chance. My book and my tales from Everest also seemed to be well received, which was evident from the sales that poured in on Amazon's German website after and during the weekend.

After the last day of the show had concluded, the Cold Avenger team and I found an Irish pub, followed later by a tiki bar in the centre of the old town. We spent the last night in Nuremberg with another company from Montana who had been at the show to push and promote their line of bear spray products.

Several drinks in, one of their sales guys, who had been on the stand next to us all weekend, began to sell me the benefits of their product. I listened intently for a few moments, as best as I could through my alcohol-induced state.

'So, if you see a grizzly approach,' he said, 'you just give a couple of quick blasts of this stuff in the bear's general direction, and he'll run off quicker than Ben Johnson when he realises he's in line for a drugs test.'

It dawned on me that he thought we had grizzly bears roaming the British countryside. I had to correct him.

'Will this work on all the ferocious hedgehogs, squirrels and bunny rabbits we have?' I asked. I don't think he appreciated the humour.

We stayed till the early hours and drank the tiki bar clean. One thing I discovered that night was that Americans sure could drink—oh, that and the fact that no matter where you go in this world, you'll always find a tiki bar; and an Irish bar, for that matter. It's true. There is even an Irish bar in Lukla, the gateway to Everest, high up in the Himalayas. I have spent many a night there.

***

Once back in the UK, I almost immediately began to slip into an almighty depression. I could feel it coming on, even in Germany, and I couldn't quite put my finger on what was causing it. I reasoned it had something to do with the fact that I still felt lost. Even four years after returning from Everest, I had still not been able to move on from the mountain. I was drifting through life with no real sense of purpose. With Everest no longer the one thing everyone associated me with, I lost who I was. My mind and my mental health began to systematically fall apart, and I felt helpless to prevent it.

For those of you who have also read my Everest book, you will know that I suffered one or two bouts of depression throughout my earlier life. I now accept that I am susceptible to depression's debilitating effects, after years of trying to deny it. I would often put the depression down to nothing more than a short bout of the blues, telling myself I would soon snap out of it. But in the spring of 2019, things felt different this time. Very different. I was about to find out how different, as I would hit the self-destruct button, sending myself and those closest to me to the very edge.

Tamara would turn 40 in June, and to celebrate, we had booked a short break to New York in April. Neither of us had been before, so we were looking forward to it. For me, it offered some respite against the internal daily battles I was having with my mental health. We went to see *King Kong* on Broadway and did all the usual tourist stuff that one does in New York. We really wanted to see *Hamilton*, the smash-hit musical that everyone raved about. We joined the queue at the box office on the morning of the show, and the ticket tout in front of us in the queue snapped up all the remaining $100 tickets for that day's performances.

'Excuse me, sir, could I take two of those tickets from you?'

'Sure,' he responded. 'That's $400.'

I was incredulous. 'What?' I snapped. 'I'm not paying you $200 per ticket when a few seconds ago they were $100.'

'Hey man, that's the way it goes,' he said. 'People on the street will.'

King Kong it was. I wouldn't have minded as much if it hadn't been for the young boy who sat directly in front of me through the whole production. All I could see was the head of the animatronic King Kong and this boy wafting his programme about behind his head, for the whole show. At one point, I told myself that if he kept doing it, I was going to knock him out. Tamara did offer to swap for the second half, which I declined. Chivalry was still alive and kicking. It was her 40th, after all.

The 9/11 memorial museum was particularly poignant, and we spent a good five hours wandering its many exhibits and memorials to the attacks. We went to the top of the Freedom Tower and took a boat cruise in the harbour to get up close with the Statue of Liberty. Pizza and coffee bars abounded, and we were never more than a block away from either. It was in a little pizzeria called Joe's Pizza in Greenwich Village that Tamara began to talk with a Latino chap, who mentioned that he was in New York with his band, Los Lonely Boys. A quick Google search revealed that they were a Grammy award-winning band. Later that night, we sat and watched them perform, after the drummer, who Tamara had been showing how to use Snap Chat, added us to their guest list. I recognised a few of their songs, too.

We skipped the Empire State Building, instead opting

for the view from the top of the Rockefeller Centre (The Top of the Rock). We were so enthralled with the daytime view, we went back at night, which was equally, if not more, impressive.

New York was great. It did the job of taking my mind away from my real-world problems. These problems, which were of my own making, were not at home waiting for me to return. I had taken them with me. I had just learned how to drown them out when I needed to.

In the summer, we took the girls away to Florida for a family holiday. We went with my friend Steve and his family. For three whole weeks, I had the most magical and amazing time. My depression stayed away the whole time I was there. The real joy for me was watching how much the girls were having the time of their lives. I genuinely thought this trip away had helped me to turn a corner. It was only when I returned home, and those familiar dark feelings began to take hold once again, that I realised I hadn't.

Work had completely dried up for me. We had been able to save up for the trip to Florida, mostly from Tamara's salary as a teacher and from what I was able to bring in. I was no longer earning money as a speaker, and a year earlier I'd sold the printing equipment that I'd used for the past 10 years to create printed clothing. Total Warrior had come to an end at the same time, so I had also lost the income that those events generated.

In the autumn of 2019, other than the monthly royalties I was earning for my Everest book, I was flat broke. I wasn't immediately concerned, as I figured that, as soon as I applied for some jobs, something would come up. With my experience, charm, good looks and all-round nice guy charisma, how could anyone say no? I had run my own company for over 10 years and had also been a motivational speaker. I felt I had a lot to offer. It was only a matter of time. Which was going to be the lucky organisation to nab me, with all my vast experience? I knew that, at this stage of my life, I was no spring chicken. I would be competing for roles against people half my age, and in some cases even younger. I'm not saying we're an ageist society, but I'm convinced I didn't get several roles I applied for because we're an ageist society. There, I've said it. Lock me up and throw away the key. I think the market for entering the workforce gets considerably harder the older you get. Even with what I assumed was a wealth of life experience and a whole raft of valuable skills and talents, I wasn't so much getting thanks as getting no thank you. It was a demoralising and soul-crushing experience. It's not even as if I was applying for positions above my station. These were basic entry-level roles I was being dismissed out of hand for. For someone as ambitious and driven as I am, it was the most scarring feeling of rejection and unworthiness I had ever felt. Even an outdoor equipment store which specialised in lightweight backpacking equipment and was a 20-minute drive from my front door didn't deem me worthy enough to have an interview for a customer service role. That was rejection on a cruel scale. I could have run the entire company, not just its customer services department.

In early autumn, I was hurting, and each job I didn't hear back from just twisted the knife that little bit more into my spine. Twelve months earlier, I'd been able to stand up on a stage and motivate a room full of accountants to be better at their jobs. And now, a year down the line, I couldn't even land a job flipping burgers—or at least, that's how it felt. I didn't apply to either of the two big burger franchises, so perhaps I'm being a bit unfair there. Note to self: must send a CV into McDonald's as soon as I've finished writing this book.

This lack of progress with job hunting would darken my

already damaged ego and pride, not to mention locking my mind further into that room in hell, reserved exclusively for me. The disdain I began to feel for myself would show no let-up. I continually compared myself to everyone around me, and it wouldn't take much to send my mind careering into the darkest of places.

For around a year, I'd investigated the possibility of offering treks to Everest Base Camp. I'd done it three times myself, so I felt this experience would stand me in good stead. I also felt the book I wrote would further cement my credentials as a viable trek leader. I still had the community on Facebook at which to target my newly launched Everest Dream Treks. I was hopeful that I would get some takers. I started to get some interest, but nothing concrete. One such taker, though, was a German lady called Andrea. She had read my book and had even been to Everest previously, but this was from the Tibetan side, after she had won a radio competition to visit the mountain for free. She had been disappointed on that trip at not being able to get close to the mountain. She had always dreamed of going back and seeing the mountain from its southern side through Nepal. She now looked to me to help her achieve that goal. Andrea had initially contacted me over a year earlier when I'd first put the feelers out about a potential trip. She was a definite solid client, and she had even filled in all the forms I had sent her, as well as offer to pay a deposit.

At one stage, a trip back to the mountain in the autumn of 2019 looked highly probable. I had taken deposits from several people, and it looked as though I would get to trek back up to the mountain with five to six individuals. But then, as often happens in my life, it started to unravel. Three members pulled out, wanting to swap for the following spring, and I had to refund deposits to two others who couldn't get the time off work required to trek to Everest.

One guy had completely misunderstood and assumed it could be done in one week. When I told him he would need three, he dropped out.

I was down to just one client, Andrea. The first person who contacted me when I first advertised the trek. Andrea was still 100 percent committed. She'd even gone as far as booking the time off work. I felt obliged to run the trip, but with just a single client I couldn't make it profitable. If anything, I would have been out of pocket. I considered running it anyway and using the experience for future marketing. Once I had been with clients, whether that was one or several, it would an easier sell for future trips, with recent experience under my belt.

Be that as it may, no matter how much I wanted this to happen and studied the viability of going, I couldn't make the maths work. I informed Andrea I had to pull the plug. I knew she would be disappointed, which she naturally was. But then she did something I wasn't expecting. She offered to up the price she'd agreed to pay me. In fact, she didn't just up it, she doubled it. There was now a real opportunity to return to the mountain—my first time back since fleeing after the earthquake four years earlier. With a single client, it would be a personal and close-knit adventure, one which Andrea was thrilled to consider.

Once more, luck would go against me. Lukla, the airstrip and gateway to Everest, had been closed most of the year to all incoming mountain flights originating out of Kathmandu. This was due to construction work, which was being carried out at Tribhuvan, the international airport at Kathmandu. The only workaround was a four-hour bus journey to a town called Ramechhap, and then hope to pick up a short mountain flight from there to Lukla, fighting against the crowds and possibly experiencing days' worth of delays. It didn't sound fun. This was a complete pain, and as far as I was concerned it was all but a showstopper. An alternative solution to this would have been to use a helicopter to fly direct to Lukla, but that would have been expensive, adding thousands of dollars to the budget. Once again, I would have been out of pocket, and it wouldn't have been fair to pass this cost on to the client—in this case, Andrea. I explained all of this to her once more in an email, informing her that if she still wanted me to guide her, I would once more need to up the price.

This was all becoming very silly, and I had no intentions of charging Andrea the now-$7,500 USD I would need for us both to helicopter into the Everest region, and for me to make a wage from the trip. I asked Andrea what the main aim was. It was for her to trek to Everest Base Camp and stand at the bottom of the mountain. She could achieve that with or without me guiding her. I told her I could organise everything for her from the moment she would land in Kathmandu airport to the moment she would get back. I would arrange for a Nepalese guide to run the trip, she would have a porter to help with bags, and I would even sort out the flight to Lukla. If I didn't go, she could afford to fly into the mountains in a helicopter and still save a few thousand dollars on what she would have had to pay to me.

Once I explained all of this to her, she was happy to take my suggestion on board. I began organising the entire trip. I booked her accommodation in Kathmandu, all the tea houses and lodges she would stay at in the mountains and booked her onto a return helicopter flight. Having been a passenger in helicopters in the Himalayas myself, this was an experience I didn't want her to miss out on. By not being there, guiding her myself, she wouldn't have to. I realised I was being selfless, but I couldn't have lived with myself If I'd taken her money, making her pay way over the odds to see the mountain. She could achieve her dream without being exploited, and I was more than happy to help her achieve it. I wondered how many other guides would have done that.

Three weeks later, Andrea achieved her dream and stood at the bottom of the mountain. She recorded herself in a very emotional video message and thanked me for helping to make her dreams come true. I couldn't help but feel a pang of sadness at not being there to share the moment with her. I regret that I didn't get to return to the mountain, but I don't regret what I did. I would do it again if ever a situation like it should re-emerge.

***

For me, my life carried on. With no income coming in, I was on very borrowed time. It was also beginning to take its toll on my relationship with Tamara. Our marriage has always been one based on strength and teamwork. Even during our most testing of times, such as the avalanche on Everest, we would come together and get through anything. This time, though, cracks were beginning to appear. The veneer that had always held us tightly together was beginning to peel away. Unless I found a job and fast, I couldn't see how we would survive.

I was sitting on the sofa in my daughters' playroom one Saturday in October. I was watching the Rugby World Cup in Japan. Ireland were playing against the New Zealand All-Blacks in a quarter-final match. There was nothing remarkable about the day. It was a cold and dreary autumn afternoon, and my daughter Isla was just pottering around somewhere, doing her own thing. My older daughter Lara had slept out at friends' the night before, so was not at home. Tamara was upstairs in the study doing some schoolwork, so I figured I would just relax in front of the TV for a few hours and watch the rugby. That is when it hit.

I have never experienced a heart attack before, so I had

no frame of reference as to what was happening. In a state of total panic, I was convinced the sudden jolt I had just experienced in my chest, followed by the crushing sensation I started to feel, was as serious as this thing could get. Convinced my heart was giving up on me, I shouted—no, wait, I screamed—for Tamara at the top of my lungs.

She frantically flew down the stairs, shouting, 'What is it? What's wrong?' In the process, she alerted Isla to the unfolding drama.

'I'm not sure,' I said, rather breathless, clutching a hand to my chest. 'I think I might be having a heart attack. You'd better call for someone.'

Tamara immediately sensed the seriousness of the situation and sprang into action, scrambling around looking for her phone. Isla began to cry and looked terrified. I tried to calm her down.

'It's okay, darling,' I said. 'Daddy will be fine. I'm just having a little trouble catching my breath right now.'

But I was far from fine, and inside I was as scared as my 10-year-old daughter looked. I wasn't ready to die, and I certainly wasn't ready to keel over and do so in my home, in front of my wife and child. Everest had done her best to take me out, a few years earlier, but hadn't succeeded. I would be damned if I were going to let something as completely random as a heart attack finish the job Everest could not.

'Pull yourself together,' I kept muttering to myself over and over. 'You're only 46, for goodness' sake. This can't be happening.'

But it was happening, or at least something was happening. I just didn't know what.

The ambulance pulled up outside my home. For the past five minutes, I'd been outside, bent over on all fours on my driveway. I was breathing in and out, counting each breath.

For some reason, I had to be outside. I didn't want to be in the house, and I didn't want to be anywhere near the room where I'd been watching the rugby. I was doing everything and anything I could think of to take my mind off the excruciating tightness I felt in my chest. My whole body was shaking.

By now, my mum had arrived. Tamara had called her after she'd called for an ambulance. She naturally looked equally as concerned and worried as Tamara did. When Tamara had called for the ambulance, the operator had advised for me to chew an aspirin tablet, which was thought to help alleviate the effects of a heart attack by stopping blood from clotting.

At this stage, it was all speculation. Even the paramedic, who had by now got me back inside the house and lying on my back on the sofa, was unsure what was causing my heart to beat out of my chest.

'Calm down,' she repeatedly told me. 'I need you calm'.

But I couldn't calm myself down. My whole body was trembling, as if in a state of shock.

The paramedic started to get a little annoyed. 'Look, Ellis,' she barked, 'unless you slow down your breathing, I can't help you.'

I eventually cottoned on to the fact that I might be bringing this on myself. My breathing began to become more regular, and the paramedics were able to get some initial tests done, blood pressure, ECG, etc. But they weren't 100 percent sure what was going on. To be on the safe side, they would take me to a hospital, where further checks could be carried out.

In the ambulance on the way, I was still convinced that I had just experienced some form of cardiac incident and was still in its grip. The intense crushing sensation would come in waves, and with each one, I also experienced a heavy, foreboding sense of doom. What the fuck was going on? None of this was normal. It felt to me like my whole body was packing in—not only my heart, but also my mind and cognitive thinking. By the time the ambulance had screeched up outside the doors to the Accident and Emergency department, I was completely out of it, not even sure where I was or even who I was anymore.

'Tell me, Ellis, have you got anything that's worrying you right now?' probed the doctor who I was now sitting naked in front of from the waist up.

My whole torso was covered in sticky electrodes from the ECG that the paramedics, and then the hospital, had carried out. With a heart attack suspected, I was seen quickly. When the occurrence of any obvious physical, medical abnormality was ruled out, the attention fell fully on the state of my mental health.

'You don't look well,' said the female doctor, before asking whether I was stressed or worried.

If ever there was a time to be honest, not only with myself but also with this perfect stranger asking if everything was okay, now was that time. This is your chance, Ellis. Accept that all's not well and get the help you need.

'No, I'm fine,' I responded. Doh! Why did I do that?

Tamara, who was in the room with me, would elaborate if she felt I wasn't being fully truthful. Even now, when being asked if all was well, I was still doing the typical man thing of trying to underplay my situation.

'I'm sure it's nothing to worry about,' I said. 'I'll snap out of it.'

These five short words would become my go-to words whenever I felt my depression was worsening. I'll snap out of it.

Tamara chimed in, 'But you've been saying that for months now, Ellis, and you haven't snapped out of it. You need help.'

It wasn't this junior cardiologist's area of expertise or her place to tell me what was wrong with me, but she knew what I had just experienced.

'There is nothing wrong with your heart. It's fine.' As soon as those words had left the doctor's lips, the sense of relief was palpable. I was informed that I had experienced a classic panic attack, with all the classic symptoms present. A heart beating out of its chest, shortness of breath, crushing pain in the chest, a sense of fear and doom. I had just suffered all that over the past few hours.

The problem with a panic attack is that there is a large crossover with several of the symptoms also present in an actual heart attack. I had never had a panic attack before in my life, ever. Why would I get one now—a middle-aged man in his forties? I didn't get it. I accepted it as the explanation, though, and was relieved at being able to leave the hospital, still with a healthy heart but also with a telephone number for a psychological service provider, who I was advised to call to make an appointment. I arrived back home, put the number in my bedside drawer and forgot all about it.

'I don't need that,' I told myself. 'I can beat this thing on my own. I'll snap out of it.'

No one could understand how I was feeling. No one. Not even Tamara. My life was playing out like one big real-life version of Instagram. Everywhere I looked, I saw people living better lives than me. Everyone seemed happy, everyone seemed so much better than me. This slowly eroded my mind, and there was nothing I could do about it. I just gave in to my fate and accepted that this was now who I was.

The four-day trip to New York in April offered me some respite, followed by the family summer holiday in

Florida. But ultimately, I could not escape from the clutches of despair, failure and unworthiness and the complete hopelessness that I felt.

There is a term used to describe the act of criticising and undermining the success and ambitions of other people. This 'Tall Poppy Syndrome,' references the notion that the 'tallest poppy' should be cut down to size. Poppies should all grow together at the same height and the same speed. If one outgrows the others, then out come the shears. This is a poisonous way to look at things and, without realising it, I was displaying tendencies leaning towards it. This culture of criticising, resenting and undermining the success of others is a highly toxic way of thinking, and one that, sadly, I had fallen foul of. I would never be openly critical of someone's else's success, but internally I began to become resentful and jealous.

To make matters worse, everywhere I looked I appeared to be surrounded by successful and happy people. Or at least, that was what my mind was telling me. From best friends, neighbours, friends of friends, Tamara's friends, Tamara's friends' husbands, those husbands' friends, the Amazon delivery driver, the school pedestrian crossing warden outside my daughters' school. Everyone had achieved more than I had in life, and everyone was gloriously happy and content. Everyone, that was, except me.

This horrific mindset began to destroy my self-esteem. I began to feel incredibly worthless, not even worthy of spending an evening socialising with friends. I simply dreaded being in a position where I would have to converse with others in a social setting. As far as I was concerned, I had failed in my life. What would I talk about if the conversation were directed my way? I had nothing to feel proud of anymore—not since my Everest trips, and they were fast becoming a distant memory.

When I look back at this now, I know the reason for this dread was caused by these completely absurd feelings of ineptitude and, I guess, by me seeing myself as a disappointment to everyone who knew me. But more so to Tamara and my mum, whom I was convinced I had let down massively. The sad irony in all of this is that some of the proudest moments of my life are the ones steeped in failure, and Everest was right up there, leading the charge. Having a dream to climb the highest mountain in the world, doing something about it and then actually trying to achieve it all ultimately ended in tragic failure. No matter how much I sugar-coated it, there was no getting away from the fact that I had failed in my endeavours. In late 2019, this was once more tearing me apart.

I felt I was destined to remain miserable for the rest of my days, yet I knew this was completely and utterly illogical. Tamara would continually tell me that all these feelings and ludicrous thoughts were just of my own making. She would tell me that no one else thought these things about me, and that she was proud of me and a lot of people thought highly of me. But here is the problem; when you have very low self-esteem, it's hard to see the wood for the trees. I knew I had a problem. I knew I had slipped back into the pit of hopelessness that is severe depression. But I didn't know what I was going to do about it.

Throughout the rest of October, into November, some days I couldn't even bring myself to get out of bed. Tamara would leave the house early; I would see the girls off to school and then I would crawl back into bed and pull the duvet over my head. I was burying my head in the sand and attempting to shut out the outside world as much as I could. It was an outside world I felt I no longer had a part in. I would send Tamara text messages, telling her I loved her and that I was sorry I had failed her. She would reply, telling me that I had not and that she and the girls loved me.

It wasn't all 24 hours, 7 days a week doom and gloom. Some days I would wake up feeling amazing. like all was right in the world again. These are what I like to call my 'Superman' days. On those days, I would get to take a break from depression's grip and don my cape. These are the times when I am most energised and focused. I wish I could say I experience lots of these days, but the truth is that I don't. For every one of those days when I feel like the Man of Steel, several will follow where it feels like I am under the debilitating effects of kryptonite.

The thing with depression is—or certainly, the thing with my depression was—the kryptonite days far outweighed the Superman days. On the days when I wasn't wearing my cape, I struggled to become enthused about pretty much anything. A ladies' volleyball team could have been parading naked outside my house, and I wouldn't even have batted an eyelid. But once I pulled on my metaphorical cape, the world suddenly became full of unlimited possibilities, with new horizons as far as the eye could see.

Of course, we cannot be happy and well-adjusted all the time. If we all spent our days as overjoyed as an eight-year-old in Disney World, how would we ever know when to be sad? When to cry? When to mourn? When to get in touch with the full range of human emotions that we have been given? We all laugh, we all cry. We all get frustrated, and we will all one day die. We can be in a great mood one day and thoroughly miserable the next. This is my 'Superman theory'. Some days we feel like Superman. Most days, we don't. Some people are positive, some people are negative. Some people can spend their entire lives on an even keel, feeling no real happy highs or low lows. And then others will spend their lives fighting the invisible battle against debilitating and completely irrational depression. Sometimes, the battle becomes too much.

Back to that day on the beach. Convinced I wanted out from the misery I was feeling daily, I drove to the beach, certain I was going to end my life. A series of things had collided to create the perfect storm of depression, which I no longer felt well enough or strong enough to continue fighting. Adjustment disorder, tall poppy syndrome, imposter syndrome, no career, no job, no future, no hope. All of it forced me into the abyss that day.

With my head under the water, spluttering for my very life, I experienced what can only be described as a flashback. I was no longer submerged in a freezing sea in the dead of winter, about to drown. I was back on Everest. It was the moment the earthquake struck, and a ton of snow began to rain down on me. Convinced I was about to die that day on Everest, through no fault of my own making, I remember feeling an incredible amount of guilt. Guilt at leaving my girls behind, leaving them without their dad. And now here I was, four years later, about to leave my girls behind yet again. This time, it would be of my making. It would be completely and emphatically 100 percent my fault. I was seconds away from shattering not only my own life but those of everyone who loved me. It wasn't fair to do this to innocent lives.

It was unfathomable, what I was prepared to do. This very vivid flashback from Everest and the sensations I'd felt at the time snapped me back from the brink. Just as I was about to succumb to the sea, I lifted my head up through the surface, spluttering and struggling to catch my breath. Ella continued to bark. I noticed two people had also strode out into the shallows and had been frantically shouting. I wasn't sure what they were saying, but I knew it was directed at me. I waded back to the shore, feeling nothing but numbness in both my mind and body. I had tried to take my own life, and I couldn't even do that.

When I reached Ella, I noticed that the two people who had been concerned for my welfare were an elderly couple who had been walking their Jack Russell terrier. It was not fair to bring this couple in on my woes, so I told them I was practising cold water immersion, which I did often. Accepting that as the likely scenario, they strode off, leaving Ella still barking and jumping up at me frantically. They say dogs can detect certain things. I am sure she knew what I was attempting to do that day. It's probably no coincidence that she's been incredibly close to me ever since.

Shivering violently, I wandered back up to my car. I left the bottle of whisky I had been swigging on the sand but grabbed my bag. I ignored everyone's concerned glances as I shuffled past, shivering uncontrollably. I switched the engine on and turned the heating up to full. I then sat there in the driving seat for a full hour, sobbing my eyes out. This was one misadventure that had been too close for comfort. I knew I needed help, and I knew that the time for that help was now. I feared that the next time this would happen, I might just succeed in doing what I set out to do. I was being a complete selfish prick; this time, I really did need to snap out of it.

When I was back home later that day, Tamara sent me a text message during one of her breaks between teaching.

'Hi gorge. How's your day going?'

This was a daily check-in from Tamara, to which I would usually send the same response back: 'I'm fine,' or something similar.

On this day, though, I responded with the following: 'I have just tried to end it all in the sea, I can't take anymore. Apart from that, I'm fine.' Even in as serious a moment as this, you could count on me to still look for the humour in any situation.

Tamara certainly didn't see the funny side. She called my friend Mark, who advised her to call a crisis team. Later that night, I had to speak over the phone to the team, to give them my permission so they could come to my house to meet me.

The following day, I sat in my dining room opposite three social workers trained to deal with situations such as this. Tamara sat by my side.

'We'll get through this,' she said.

Every day for the next two weeks, a member of the team would come out to my house and meet me, concerned that I may still do something reckless. They needed to be certain that I wouldn't before they would discharge me to psychological services. Every day I was told I was ill, and that it was nothing to feel ashamed or embarrassed about. I was compared to being everything from a broken-down boiler to a high-speed performance sports car. They can both break down, and they both need servicing. I was asked by one of the social workers who visited one day: if I broke my arm, would I wear a cast?

When I responded that of course I would, she said, 'Well, that's what we're doing with your brain. It's currently a bit broken, so we're preparing a cast for it to help it heal.'

I seriously hoped she wasn't being serious. I couldn't imagine wearing a cast around my head. I certainly didn't want to wander around looking like Beavis from Beavis and Butt-Head.

During those two weeks, I was visited by several individuals, who all sat intently and listened to my story. For the first time in my life, I was speaking openly to strangers about how I was feeling. A huge weight was being lifted. I felt like I was finally on the road to recovery. Would I finally leave this room from hell? I very much hoped so, even though I knew it wouldn't happen overnight.

When I was finally discharged, I was placed on a waiting list, to begin a course of counselling. I would begin that counselling at the start of 2020, where I would spend several sessions with a therapist, who helped me to understand more about what had been going on with my life. It all came down to adjustment disorder and loss of purpose in my life. At the end of the sessions, I was convinced I knew what I wanted to do for the rest of my life. I didn't care what I did, as long as I was able to give back. I wanted to help people. To do that, I needed to be able to help people. I needed to look after myself before I could help anyone else.

That Christmas, I suffered several more panic attacks, but at least I knew the signs and knew what was happening. We had gone across to Cumbria for Christmas, sharing a large estate on the edge of the Lake District with Tamara's sister and family and around 20 other people, whom we had never met. My anxiety at having to speak to people and possibly having to tell them what I did for a living went through the roof. However, I managed to keep it in check. To think just over a year earlier, I was being paid to be a confident, self-assured, inspirational public speaker. Now, the thought of having to communicate with someone I didn't know reduced me to a quivering nervous wreck.

That week away was well needed, and despite a minor blip on the night of Christmas Eve, when I was once again convinced I was having a heart attack, everything else went smoothly. I even called the NHS 111 service that night and was about to get Tamara to drive me 30 miles to the nearest hospital in Keswick, at 10.00pm on Christmas Eve, where I could be seen. Luckily, I came to my senses and realised it was once more a panic attack. Poor Tamara. I had certainly kept her on her toes of late.

I needed to learn to trust myself. I had survived a hell of a lot in my life so far. I was confident I could now cope with whatever else was coming my way.

As the end of the year was approaching, I was sick and tired of staring at the four walls within my room from hell. I was ready to leave. This time I had a key, and I could unlock the door. All I had to do was insert it and twist, and I would be free. That room from hell could go fuck itself. The following year, 2020, was going to be my year. It would be an amazing year. Of that I was confident.

Whoops!

Note to self: Never be openly confident about anything again. Ever!

CHAPTER NINE
MY REINCARNATION

'There are far, far better things ahead than
anything we leave behind.'
C.S. Lewis

'Hello, Ellis!' So, tell me, how have things been with
yourself these past few weeks?' Gillian enquired over the
phone.

Since the start of the year, I had been meeting her
fortnightly to discuss and work through the horror show
that had been the previous three to four months. Gillian
was a wellbeing counsellor for Alliance Psychological
Services, a Teesside-based provider of counselling and
therapies. I had spent several hours in her company and felt
at ease discussing everything I felt had contributed towards
my rapid decline and attempted suicide. This was our last
session, and due to the COVID 19 pandemic, we had to do
it over the phone.

I was in a much better place, mentally, physically and
psychologically. While I had been facing down my demons
the previous autumn, I had all but stopped exercising. This
was very unusual for me. Usually, not a day would pass
without me flinging a kettlebell around or getting outside
for a run. When I started my therapy sessions, I began to
run again, and I felt a million percent better as a result.
Being outdoors in the cool winter air did wonders for my

state of mind, and together with the actual sessions with Gillian, this natural form of therapy undoubtedly helped to restore the equilibrium in my mind.

I could feel my entire body and mind beginning to heal and repair themselves. I had been prescribed a course of anti-depressants, but I couldn't bring myself to take them. I eventually relented and took them for a few months, but only a mild dose. When I was confident, I didn't need them anymore I stopped taking them.

I was slowly beginning to turn my life around and head in the right direction. I was running more miles per week than I had done when I had been training for Everest. The excess Christmas weight soon began to drop away. I knew I was determined to introduce a fitness regime back into my life, as I had even gone out for a long run in Cumbria on Christmas Day.

Things were starting to feel semi-normal again. I still didn't have a job or career and was therefore not creating any kind of financial platform for myself. My Everest book was still (remarkably, three years after its release) selling reasonably well. This gave me a monthly royalty cheque, which amounted to nothing more than pocket money, but as the saying goes, it was better than nothing, and it was keeping the metaphorical wolves at bay.

The Everest Dream group on Facebook was still growing and thriving, and so to bolster this online community further, I created a website through the online shopping platform Shopify. This would enable me to create designs once more and then sell those designs on physical products. I no longer had any printing equipment, but I didn't need it. There were dozens of print-on-demand suppliers I could choose to partner with. They would print and ship all the products on my behalf. I could just sit back, do nothing and cream all the profits in. Well, that was the theory behind it. But still, it was worth a shot, so I spent a few weeks creating the store and populating it with my Everest Dream product line. These products included everything from T-shirts and hoodies through to phone cases, coffee mugs and headwear. I could even offer greetings cards and canvas prints. It seemed so much easier than the old way of doing things. The only drawbacks to this new way of selling were much fewer profits and longer timeframes for delivering to customers.

What with my book, the new products and the potential to return to Nepal and trek back to the mountain, the year had started with much promise and optimism. My mind was once more alive with the buzz of positivity and prospects for the future—a future which I would be alive to see.

Around this time, I had seen a quote online from a US author/blogger by the name of Jeanette Coron. I had saved it as the wallpaper on my phone so that I'd see it every time I picked my phone up.

'Everybody goes through difficult times, but it is those who push through those difficult times who will eventually become successful in life. Don't give up, because this too shall pass.'

I immediately related to the words, and the quote became my go-to pick me up if I started to feel a little down. I was adamant that I had kicked that room from hell out of my life forever. I was sure that I would never stare at its door again.

'I will be successful in this life; I will be successful in this life. I will be successful in this life.' If I say it three times, it's more likely to happen. Like the way Beetlejuice would appear if you said his name out loud three times. I would say this mantra to myself over and over every morning I woke up and then spend 10 minutes quietly meditating.

I hadn't been able to bring myself to return to that beach

(as this book goes to print, I still haven't), so instead I opted to take Ella to another beach, near my house. Each morning I would run along the beach, with my faithful companion by my side, grateful to be alive.

Life was good again, at last. The weather was getting warmer, the nights were getting shorter and spring was in the air. My flip-flops and shorts had even come back out. I hadn't had a negative thought for months. Even critical reviews of my book were no longer stinging with the usual ferocity. 'Ah, someone else who thinks I'm a selfish prick.' They are just words on a screen, at the end of the day, I recall thinking. Sticks and stones.

The opportunities to be outside, in nature, whether that be at the beach, the local park, or quite simply wandering around my neighbourhood, made my soul sing. Shakespeare was most definitely correct when he said, 'The earth has music for those who listen.'

But then someone in China ate a bat. A virus began to spread. Our government spoke. 'Everyone inside for the next three months, please.' Welcome to 2020.

Clearly, it's not as simplistic as that. How the virus started, I guess we will never know for sure. Whether it was indeed passed from a bat, a pangolin, or another animal to a human at a seafood market in Wuhan or was created in some secret laboratory is now very much a moot point. We will leave the scientists to discover the how! As human beings living on planet earth in 2020, we have all had to deal with the now.

**

The first global pandemic lockdown began for me, as it did for most people in the United Kingdom and around the world, at the end of March.

Being able to walk Ella, our Labradoodle, around the neighbourhood every day during our allocated hour of exercise in the spring sunshine became a real joy. Just Tamara, our two daughters Lara, and Isla and I treading the same paths every day. Total bliss. But doing the same walk during the second national lockdown later that year, in November … Now that was a whole different kettle of fish.

'Lara, Isla, come on. We're going out with the dog. Get your jackets, hats, scarf, gloves, wellies and facemask on.'

We're going for a walk. Queue the backlash.

'Do we have to, Dad?' they would say every night after school. 'It's freezing and it's dark,' or, as Lara dared say one night after becoming a bit braver with her resistance, 'It's bloody freezing!'

'Yes, you do. Now hurry up and get ready to go. We're leaving in five, and watch your language, young lady.'

Being outside in the fresh air is a fundamental human right. Luckily, governments around the world realised that, knowing the benefits to mental health that the outdoors can bring. Outside is outside, no matter where you are or what you are going through, or what the world is going through, whether on the side of a mountain, running along a sandy beach, or taking a night-time stroll around your local park during a global pandemic. I urge everybody to get outside if you are feeling glum. Just don't try and drown yourself in a cold sea in the depths of winter.

Tamara would often tell me how she thought I would make a great teacher. It was her profession, and I had considered it fleetingly, but ultimately, I'd never done anything about it.

One day into the New Year, she said, 'I'm serious. Why don't you think about it?'

Before the pandemic and the resulting imminent lockdown, I would give it some serious thought. I knew I would make a good teacher—a fantastic teacher, if I'm being honest. And yes, I am blowing smoke up my arse.

Three years of visiting schools as a speaker had shown me that I had a talent and an innate ability to engage and communicate effectively with school-age children. The less said about my stint as a life-skills coach, the better. Being a failure at my education during my school days has always been a blight and a deep regret in my life. I didn't get the grades in my exams at age 16 that would have propelled me onto further education, better job prospects and a good all-round grounding as a young adolescent. It haunts me to this day.

To train to become a teacher in the UK, you need to possess three things: a bachelor's degree, check; a GCSE pass in English, uncheck; a GCSE pass in Maths, again uncheck. One out of three wasn't bad. I had the most difficult part of the qualifying trio, the degree. If I were serious about training to become a teacher, I would need to address the other two missing items, namely the Maths and English grades.

My problem with teaching was never lacking the ability to teach, it was always what subject I would teach. During the conversation with Tamara that day, I decided that Computer Science was to be my chosen subject if I were to go through with this. This was down to a couple of deciding factors. Firstly, computers are the future; everyone knows that. Secondly, it was the subject that Tamara taught. Tamara would have all the teaching resources and lesson plans I would need; therefore, I wouldn't need to actually plan any lessons or work. That sounded great. But lastly, and possibly most significantly of all the factors in choosing computing as my area of expertise, it paid a £28,000 tax-free bursary for the year. I could earn while I was learning. I did consider Geography, but the bursary for this subject was significantly less. Computer Science it was.

Shortly before the lockdown kicked in, I attended an

interview at the training school affiliated to the school Tamara worked at. I sat a written assessment and taught a killer lesson on an introduction to binary to a room full of 11-year-olds, thanks to Tamara and her amazing slides. In the actual face to face interview with the head of the school, I gave several compelling reasons why I would make a great teacher at this stage of my life. I was duly offered a place on the course, starting in September, providing I resat the papers in Maths and English. Finally, everything in my life was working out, for once. All I had to do was get through lockdown and a UK summer and pass two school-level exams before beginning my new career as a member of the teaching profession. You know what they say; those that can't, teach.

With the lockdown in full effect and a pandemic sweeping the nation, I couldn't allow myself to drift aimlessly. Trekking back to Everest was once more off-limits, with the travel restrictions imposed. Companies were laying off and furloughing staff members left, right and centre, and finding a job during a national lockdown was not going to be easy.

Tamara worked from home during this time, teaching her lessons online. With all the schools closed, the girls were at home too, being home-schooled. I used the time to study up on computer science and revise to pass the two exams, in Maths and English.

I have never been one of those individuals who believes you should have no regrets in life. How can anyone get through this life and not have any regrets? I have a lot of regrets, built up from a life of mishap, strife and adventure. 'Never regret yesterday. Life is in you today and you make your tomorrow.'– L. Ron Hubbard.

I know what you're thinking right now. Did Ellis just quote the founder of Scientology to prove some convoluted point he's trying to make? Yes, I did. Stick with me on this.

I have never bought into that way of looking at things. You might be the founder of Scientology, Mr Hubbard, but I think you are wrong. I think it is perfectly natural to have regrets in life. After all, how are we supposed to grow and correct our mistakes if we regret nothing? I regret not asking out Jenny, a girl I fancied at school when I was 13 years old. I regret painting my first ever car, a Ford Escort XR3, with a tin of black masonry paint. I regret breaking into a paper factory when I was in my teens with a group of friends and then scattering thousands of Post-it notes around the streets of the town. I regret that I didn't get to climb high on Everest. I regret that I never got to see the northern lights in Iceland. I regret that I have never been stoned on cannabis and then danced naked in the rain.

Those last three regrets I could potentially do something about.

You see, it's perfectly acceptable to have regrets. You should regret lots in life and attempt to rectify those that bother you the most. Overall, I don't regret the things I've done. I just regret the things I didn't do when I should have, like passing my GCSEs in English and Maths when I was 16 years old. I wish, looking back, that I could have got hold of that unruly little shit and hammered some sense into him.

'Yes, Ellis—sorry, Stuart—your exams really do matter, and unless you do something about it now to correct this, you will always regret it. And here, while we are at it; have a fist in the face. Pow!'

Hopefully, then, a bloodied younger version of myself would have wiped away the blood from his nose, heeded that advice and done something about it. Then present-day Ellis would not be having to consider going back to school, aged 46 and ¾, to pass school leaver standard exams to become a teacher. What a schmuck!

By becoming a teacher, what did I have to lose, and what was the worst that could happen? Nothing, right? Pass those exams, and it was in the bag. My new vocation as a teacher could begin.

It was for this reason that I found myself at home during the first COVID-19 lockdown, revising to pass my school exams in Maths and English, 30 years after I should have passed them the first time.

***

In this book of misadventure, throughout the many trials and tribulations of my life, I have been visited many times by the misadventure fairies. I couldn't possibly reach the end of this book without another visit from those supernatural, mythical little fuckers. This time, they really would mess things up for me.

A few days into the summer holidays, I received a call from the head of the training school, asking me if I would attend a meeting the following morning with her and the head of the entire education trust that the training school was part of.

'Sure,' I said. 'Is everything okay?'

'We'll discuss it in the morning. See you tomorrow.'

It was a warm summer's day. I turned up for the meeting, doing my best to look like a windswept Australian surf dude, with my scraggly thick beard, baggy cargo shorts, flip-flops, AC/DC T-shirt and sunglasses clipped to the top of my head. What was I thinking? I know this wasn't a formal interview, but I should have done better than this. I have to say, this is a look I have cultivated and perfected from years of not having to conform to societal demands. In almost 20 years of working for myself, I have never had to answer to anyone, nor dress to impress anyone other than myself. Even on my Facebook profile at the time, I described myself as a tie-loathing adventurer and underachiever. I truly live by the mantra that life is better in flip-flops, and unfortunately for me, I chose the wrong meeting and the wrong individual on whom to exercise that conviction.

As I sat down in front of the head of the education trust, I still didn't have a clue why I was there. It didn't take me long to realise that, for whatever reason I was there that day, things weren't going to end well.

After a quick glance up and down, it was obvious that this lady had taken an instant dislike to the way I'd turned up. The first words out of her mouth confirmed as much.

'I haven't met you before, and I had nothing to do with your interview and selection for the course, but had I done so, I would probably not have offered you a place.'

Holy shit! Just what had I done to offend this individual so quickly? Maybe she didn't like AC/DC. Her next probing line of interrogation revealed all.

'Why did you conceal information from your application form?' she asked. 'You do realise you have committed fraud?'

'I'm sorry? Say what, now?'

Apparently, on the application form I had filled in when applying for the training course, in the section where it asked me if I had a criminal conviction, I had ticked the box for 'no', as I wrongly believed I didn't have any criminal convictions. But the background check the trust had carried out on me revealed that I did, unbeknownst to me.

I sat nervously in my seat, shifting uncomfortably at what was about to be revealed about my delinquent history, wondering what I had done and if I should have a solicitor present. I was genuinely curious as to what I could have done. It was most definitely nothing significant, or I would have known about it and declared it—whatever 'it' was.

She leaned across her table and spun the enhanced disclosure certificate she had in my name around so I could read it. She pointed to the part she wanted me to see.

Conviction Details

Date of Conviction: 10 December 1993

Offence: Making a False Statement or representation
to obtain benefit or payment on social security
administration act 1992.

Fine: £75.00

Costs: £65.00

In the early 90s, I'd worked as a nightclub DJ. I was
19 years old, fresh out of a college course in swimming
pool management. I naturally put the course to good use
by opting instead to earn some money spinning records
several nights a week. I wasn't very good at it, and it was
no surprise that I didn't last very long in the profession. I
ended up being fired (surprise, surprise) one New Year's
Eve when I showed up for work late and seven sheets to the
wind. When I eventually made it to the club, over two hours
late and stinking of cheap cider, the manager told me to
sling my hook. It was a fair one. I didn't argue. And that was
that. Or so I thought!

A few months later, they called me back to ask if I could
cover a few shifts to get them out of a jam, as their new
club DJ was sick. I figured I owed them, so I agreed to
help. I ended up working several shifts in the full glare of
a nightclub. The only difference this time around was the
fact that, a few months earlier, I had signed on to claim
unemployment benefit due to being fired from the job. I

didn't bother informing the benefits office of this extra income, as I figured it was only temporary and not worth their time knowing about it. Unfortunately, somebody decided it was worth them knowing about it and decided to let them know. To this day, I have no idea who, or even why.

A month later, I had a date in court, where I was made to pay back the £75 fine and the £65 in costs. I was made an example of and even had my name plastered over the local press, with the headline 'DJ in Benefits Fiddle.' I was mortified. Once again, I had made the front cover of the local newspaper, and once again it was for unsavoury reasons, just as, when I was a small boy, I had climbed onto the roof of that chapel.

As I sat there that day, with my entire teaching career unravelling before it had even begun, a petty incident from 26 years ago, which I had forgotten about, had come back to seal my fate. I had a criminal conviction that I hadn't declared; therefore, I had committed deception and lied on my application, and therefore they couldn't let me commence the course, therefore it was the end of my teaching career. Therefore, thank you, but no thank you.

I defended myself as best as I could, but I could see my protestations were falling on deaf ears. I had been accused of a crime, found guilty and sentenced, all in the amount of time it took for me to sip my bottle of water.

I took my sorry self and my AC/DC T-shirt and left the office. Then it hit me. Oh, no! What was I going to tell Tamara? This was my wife's employer, at the end of the day, and they had just fired a colleague's husband. They could have given me the benefit (excuse the pun) of the doubt. I didn't lie. I am sure, if pushed on the issue, the trust would have said they didn't have a choice. But they did. Everyone has a choice. They just chose not to exercise it, for whatever reason. I blame that AC/DC T-shirt.

When you look at the reasons why some things in life don't work out, you must take on board a level of personal responsibility. Ultimately, I wouldn't become a teacher because I failed to declare a piece of information. Although petty and trivial and no worthier than a parking ticket, in my eyes, it was a big deal to them. I had used deceit and not been truthful on an official document, and it had cost me everything.

When I now look back, I think teaching didn't work out for me because I didn't want it enough. Sometimes, the universe will jump in and lend a hand if it thinks you're about to make a mistake. With teaching, I would have made a big mistake. It was never my profession. It was my wife's. I considered it at a time in my life when options on the table were severely limited. All I had to do during the lockdown and the summer was revise and pass two exams, in Maths and English. But at the time of the meeting that sealed my fate, I still hadn't sat the exams. I had kept putting them off until the very last date possible. I think this lack of commitment to the cause must have been evident to see.

In this life, I like to believe that certain things happen for a reason. This was not the path I was meant to go down. At the time, I thought the decision to remove me from the course was harsh, but I now look at it differently. I had been spared from starting a career that my heart and soul were not committed to. I would have been a great teacher; I am not disputing that. But my calling was elsewhere, outside the classroom, away from teaching 12-year-olds how to use spreadsheets and code programming languages, neither of which I could do anyway.

***

As an interesting note to the above events, on the same day my teaching career was unravelling around me, after being deemed unworthy, I was being honoured in my daughter's primary school. The school gave out a new annual award to one of its pupils which was to recognise commitment and achievement in sporting or other extra-curricular activities. This was a huge honour. Due to the pandemic, I wasn't able to attend in person to present the inaugural award to a year 5 girl, who was a gifted athlete. But I was asked to record a short video. On the award, itself which was a solid statute of glass which resembled a block of ice, the following inscription was etched;

'The Stewart Aspirational Award for Outstanding Achievement and Aiming High – Awarded to a child who knows the best view comes after the hardest climb.'

Have I said yet, that life moves in mysterious ways? My life certainly does.

With my little teaching misadventure out of the way, I was back at square one. But this time, square one excited me. When I finished the therapy at the start of the year, I was convinced my true calling in life was to try to help people and to give back. That was what counted the most to me. Everest Dream on Facebook was a platform where I could do this, to an extent. If someone should post a comment seeking advice on the base camp trek or another aspect of the mountain I was familiar with, then I would answer as best I could. Speaking to others about the mountain was thankfully something I had gained a lot of practice of, not just from my days as a speaker, but also from responding to the many positive comments I would regularly receive about the book.

I have always responded whenever someone has taken time out of their day to contact me regarding my Everest book. I have received the most heart-warming and wonderful messages since it was published four years ago. It appears my book has motivated, inspired and educated thousands of readers. Sometimes those readers reach out to me and let me know how grateful they are to me for writing it. I received a particularly heartfelt and emotionally charged email from a chap a few years back, who said my book had helped to save his life. He said after reading *It's Not About the Summit* that he'd realised almost anything was possible in life.

I would be lying if I said these comments and other similar messages didn't make me feel proud. Of course they did. As the author of a book, it's always nice to think it can have a meaningful and positive impact on the reader. With the Everest book, I know I attained that. For that reason, it is one of the proudest achievements of my life to date.

In September 2020, news emerged that Doug Scott, the first Brit to climb Everest and whose boot shed I had tidied up five years earlier, was gravely ill and had been since the beginning of the UK's first lockdown. Doug who was now 79, had been diagnosed with cerebral lymphoma, a cancer of the brain, which sadly was inoperable. Community Action Nepal, the charity Doug had founded over 20 years previously, had organised a special Mount Everest Challenge in his honour. The charity was calling on people to become involved. The challenge was simple, even to those who had never stepped foot on a mountain before. All you had to do was climb your staircase 20 times and then take a photo of yourself at the 'summit' on your 20th climb. You then uploaded the photo to social media and donated. The charity patron, Chris Bonington, and one of the trustees, Paul 'Tut' Braithwaite, had thrown their full weight behind endorsing the challenge. On the 25th September, it would be 45 years since the historic first ascent of the south-west face of Everest, when Bonington had led the expedition there. Tut Braithwaite was also a member, along with Doug and several other leading climbers of the time. I wanted to become involved and do something to help, but I didn't want to just climb my stairs. But what else could I do to show my appreciation to someone who had been a big inspiration in my life? Then it hit me.

In 2015, after the earthquake that had killed thousands across Nepal and displaced people from their homes, I had created a limited-edition T-shirt which raised over $5,000. That money went directly to the families of some of the Sherpa victims who were killed on Everest when the earthquake struck. After seeing the news about Doug, I put my creative skills to good use and worked on a new design which I would then look to sell through my Everest website and community on Facebook. This design would honour the members of the 1975 South West Face Expedition and would feature several of the team members' names as part of the design. When I was happy with the finished design, I put the feelers out by posting the T-shirt on my social media channels. Within a few hours, I had generated a few sales, so I knew I was onto something.

Throughout the rest of the month, I sold over 200 of the T-shirts to people all over the UK and even to the US and Australia. I closed the campaign down on the evening of the 25th, to coincide with the anniversary of the climb. CAN that night showed a live stream on YouTube of the film *Everest: The Hard Way*. I joined in the stream and sold another 20 T-shirts while the film was being shown. I gave all the proceeds to the charity. This was more than I would have raised from sponsors if I had climbed my stairs, but I still felt I could do more.

My Everest book was sold exclusively through Amazon, but I had also sent them over 150 of my copies, which I had left from the short speaking tour I had done in 2018.

These books had hardly sold, as Amazon had pushed and promoted their copies of my book. I was competing against myself and paying storage fees for doing so. Right there, right then, I knew what I needed to do. I requested back all 155 copies of the book they were storing. When they arrived a few days later, I offered them up for sale, with all proceeds going to the charity. They sold out within a few days. It was good to know that, rather than have those books sitting around collecting dust in an Amazon warehouse, the money from their sale could now be used to benefit the mountain folk of the high Himalayas. I took a sense of pride from it, and it felt amazing. When it came to the mountain and Nepal, I still had a pull factor, and I was able to tap into it to good effect.

Although my adventures in Nepal had been five years earlier, I was still full of so much love and positivity for the country, it's people and its mountains, no matter how deadly those mountains could be. They were still stunning, and so were Nepal's people, who, during the pandemic, needed our help more than ever.

Doug Scott sadly succumbed to his cancer and died in December 2020, leaving a legacy of a life well-lived.

A year on from my darkest hour, I have reached a point in my life where I feel I am beginning to learn what I need to do to make my life well-lived.

I know who I am, and I know who I am not. I don't need a job title to define that identity. I know what drives me, what motivates me, and I now know what crushes my soul and darkens my mind. I know in my heart of hearts that I will never revisit that day at the beach. I have come through the experience, and I firmly feel this time I have emerged on the other side a stronger and more resilient individual.

I wrote this book during one of the worst years that any of us will likely ever live through. Years like this one are seldom experienced, and I very much hope we don't see another of its kind for a long time to come. However, personally, it was not my *annus horribilis*. That was the year before.

It's time to stand up and be counted among equals. I am no worse than anyone else, and I am no better than anyone else. I am just me, Ellis.

When it comes to people, there will always be those far worse off than you and I, and there will be those apparently far better off. But what does 'better off' mean?

To answer that, we should look at what 'better' means. A quick Google search brings up' more desirable, satisfactory, or effective'. Even that is ambivalent. So, your neighbour has a brand-new Range Rover parked on their driveway. According to Google, and the classic definition of what 'better' means, your neighbour is now more effective and satisfactory than you. Does having a shiny new Range Rover make them more desirable?

Does 'better' mean richer? Does it mean driving a better car, living in a bigger house? Does 'better' mean being famous? Does it mean being able to bench press 200kg or run 100 metres in 9.6 seconds? Is that the definition of 'better'? Or if someone is physically more attractive than you, does that make that person better?

Here's a newsflash for you. It doesn't.

None of that stuff matters.

And how do I know that?

Because I lived a period of my life thinking everybody was better than I was. When I was at my lowest ebb, I had convinced myself that I was on the bottom rung on the ladder of life. No matter what I did, or where I went, I could not break away from that bottom rung, and that bottom rung was a worthless place to be. I was sick of gazing up at everyone else higher up that ladder than me. Everyone was better than me. Thinking I would be trapped forever on that rung sent my mind spiralling towards a living hell. A hell created of my own doing. I had checked myself in, and only I could check out. I very nearly stayed permanently.

We live in a world that is driven by this notion of being better. Be bigger, be braver, be richer, be faster, be more confident, be bolder, be cleverer, be better looking, be more successful, be good at Instagram filters, be this, be that … It's all bullshit. The only thing you need to be is you. We need to stop chasing down expectations about what it means to be better. If, by being you, you start to achieve better things, then great. But you don't need to be consumed by it.

Being better and being successful are also two very different things. There is nothing wrong with wanting to be successful in life; surely we all want that. Being successful doesn't mean being able to buy a big house and an expensive sports car, although if you live in a mansion and drive an Aston Martin, then well done you. Being successful, in my eyes, means being happy and content. Being happy with what you have, and content with you who you are. Having more 'Superman' days than kryptonite ones.

Since I admitted I had a problem and sought the help I desperately needed, my days have been a lot more superhero than villain. My cape now gets worn more often than not.

A year ago, I would not have been able to sit down and write this book. Depression's tight chokehold had me pinned to the ground. Writing this book, or writing about any aspect of my life, was as far away from my mind as it

251

was possible to be. I was in a battle for my very survival.

The decision to produce this book happened on the toss of a dice. I'm being serious. I made a pact with myself that I would only look to write it based on the outcome of a dice toss. I gave myself the least favourable odds, too. If it lands on a six, I'll begin writing. Anything else, then I won't. The rest is history. That dice has been sitting on my desk the whole time I wrote the book, the six black dots still upright and still showing me that the universe wanted me to write.

As you have now seen, a lot of things in my life have not always panned out the way I had hoped they would. I have lived my fair share of adventure, and equally, I have experienced a large amount of misadventure, enough to last another lifetime. Parts of my life have often been chaotic and calamitous, and at times it seems as though I have not been following any conventional pathway. Unpredictability has ensued more often than not.

In writing this book, I wanted to take you on the journey that I have endured since my Everest attempts, as well as fill in some of the blanks from my earlier years.

'Endured' is a strong, and possibly a strange, choice of word to describe the past five years of my life. But it is a word which a lot of emotion can be attached to. To endure is to imply survival, suffering and a lived experience. To that end, it is the perfect way to encapsulate a life recently spent in purgatory. Endured and survived should be my new tattoo, but possibly in Latin.

Yes, I do have a tattoo. I have an unfinished tattoo. I had it done on my first visit to Kathmandu, 21 years ago. Back then, I was 26 years old, with the world laid out before me. I had fallen in love with Nepal and the whole notion of one day wanting to climb its highest mountain, so much so that I decided I should give myself a permanent reminder so I wouldn't forget. I now proudly have the Nepalese word

'Sagarmatha', which is an old Sanskrit word meaning 'peak of heaven', on my right shoulder. I vowed that, once I had stood on the top of that peak of heaven, (Everest) I would add the date. I am still waiting to add that date, despite trying twice, hence why it's an unfinished design.

With this book of misadventure, I wanted to show you what has made me the person I am today. I have made no attempt to sugar-coat any aspect of my life. What you have read is real. Every bit of it happened how I described it. Real life is raw, and it is often unadulterated and unfiltered. You can't shy away from that, and I have made no attempt to do so. The misadventures of my life have been the accidents, the mishaps and the mischance. The misfortunes I have encountered can happen in the most inconspicuous of ways as part of the overall drudgery of life. There has been nothing outwardly remarkable about any aspects of my life, but to me, I feel I have lived a remarkable life. Are we not all remarkable in our own little way?

As I stated from the outset, we all have stories to tell. Some of us will choose never to tell those tales, keeping them locked away forever, destined never to reveal those skeletons hiding away in your closet. But some of us do decide to reveal them, warts and all. I hope you will all be kind to me for doing so.

When I wrote and shared my Mount Everest story, I unintentionally opened my life to anyone who picked up a copy of the book and read it. Some of the feedback I received suggested that I had been very revealing and honest. I think that is what a good story should be, truthful and illuminating. In keeping with that tradition and in remaining true to how I tell my stories, I hope I have been able to achieve that with this book.

Sitting down during the lockdown months of 2020 and beginning to type the first few tentative words to what would become this book, I doubted very much whether I would see it through to a conclusion. I initially and wrongly dismissed huge aspects of my life, thinking they wouldn't be relevant or interesting to you, the reader. After all, who am I? I'm not a celebrity. I'm not famous for being or doing anything of note. But then, I don't need to be. Nobody does. You don't need to be famous to tell your story.

There is a strong chance that you could be reading this book, not having the faintest idea of who I am. If that is the case, then well done me. I have succeeded with this book. I have proved that you do not need to be a household name to make someone interested in reading your story. I am neither famous nor particularly talented, yet here we are.

That doesn't mean that I haven't had moments where I've had to take a step back and ask myself what I was doing. I've had to argue with the little negative voice in my head on numerous occasions.

'Why are you writing this? Who are you hoping will read it? Why are you revealing some very dark personal moments of your life?'

These are all valid questions I have asked myself. On the occasions when I couldn't find answers that would do justice to this self-interrogation, I would stop writing and take myself off to do something else, such as walking the dog or going for a run. Once I was sure I had found the answers, I would silence the voice in my head and get back to it.

I am writing this because I want other people to know that it's okay to not be okay. I hope, for everyone who reads these words, that you come to see that it's okay to screw up. It's okay not to feel normal from time to time, and it's okay to fail.

Throughout my life, the many interactions I have enjoyed with people are the essence of my existence. If you go back and read this whole book again, you will see that all the stories I have described would be nothing without some of the many interesting characters I have encountered along the way. A lot of people I have met over the years have gone on to leave some form of an impression, good or bad. Whether that be the likes of Rob Metcalfe and Tony Frobisher, whose stories of courage and bravery have inspired me beyond words, or people like Doug Scott, who motivated me to aim high. Dave Price, the coach of the dragon boat team, became my first role model when I was in my early 20s. He was one of the very first individuals I met who got me to believe more in myself.

I am who I am today because of the people I have met, and the experiences we have shared. To every passenger I picked up in my time as a taxi driver and to every person I stood up in front of and inspired with my Everest stories, these all go towards making up the foundations of my life.

Without all these experiences and interactions that we experience in our lives, I would not be me, and you would not be you.

My life has been as colourful as they come. I have made mistakes, and I have collected regrets. I try to learn from those mistakes and correct the regrets almost every day. We don't like admitting that we regret anything, because that implies we have experienced failure. And failure is a sign of weakness. As soon as you can tell yourself that it's okay to regret something, you will start to own those regrets. That is a sign of strength. Telling yourself you have never failed at anything and regret nothing is a slippery slope to a life of narcissism and selfishness. Be true to yourself and be honest with yourself.

This book is the most honest appraisal of my life to date. My weaknesses are there for all to see. By exposing my life in this manner, I have gained more strength, courage and belief in my future self than I ever thought possible.

I don't know what my future holds. I still feel young and ambitious enough to become successful one day. That success will be determined by me. I don't need to obtain a set of values to match the ideals as laid out by popular culture. I don't feel as though I am successful yet. I am much happier, and I am now much closer to contentment than I have been in recent times, but by my yardstick, I haven't yet reached the level of success I seek.

We create our opportunities in this life. And we either live or die, sink or swim based on the chances we take and the choices we make. I have always lived by the belief that I am my own life coach. No one truly knows what goes on inside your head. Only you can drive towards your destiny. After all, who knows you better than yourself?

And remember, it's okay to regret, and failure need not define you. If you remember nothing else from this book, please remember that.

Go forth and keep creating your stories. There may be adventure involved, there may be a misadventure. It doesn't matter, as long as you keep creating the stories of your life and keep the momentum going.

It is the standing still and burying our heads in the sand where the danger lies. There are crabs, and they will pinch hard.

Love,
Ellis

EPILOGUE

I haven't been able to visit 'that beach' since 'that day'. I know I will again one day, but for now, I am comfortable giving it a wide berth. It is a shame I haven't returned yet because, as far as beaches go, this one is as good as they come. With its rugged cliffs, hidden caves and dramatic seas, there is something wild and untamed about it. Which is probably why I gravitated towards it so much. There has always been something wild and untamed about me.

Before that day I had often ran along that beach, explored its caves and strolled along its long pebble and rock-strewn sands with Tamara, the girls and Ella. It was my happy place. Beaches and the sea tend to make me reflective and dreamy. If ever I felt the stresses of modern life beginning to build up, a quick drive to the beach solved everything—before it no longer did.

It's not the only coastal area near my home. I have since relocated my happy place a few miles up the coast, to a busier and more easily accessible beach.

On a recent visit, I noticed a person in the sea. Nothing unusual about that, except this was November. My mind immediately wandered back one year. Same time of year, the same sea, same weather. I wondered if this person in the water was struggling as I had been. Not battling against the cold and the tide but grappling to stay afloat in life.

I approached the shoreline with Ella but could see that this man seemed to be fine. There was no struggle taking place. I didn't need to leap into the currents to perform a gallant and heroic rescue mission. I watched for a few more moments before he began to re-emerge and walk to the shore. All he wore was a pair of swim shorts, nothing else. Brave man, I thought.

Last year I was just an idiot who didn't care what happened when I strode into that sea. This person appeared to be dipping into the sea purely for recreation. I had to speak to him to find out why.

'Hi. Bruce. Nice to meet you,' he said, after I had jokingly enquired if he was mad.

It turns out Bruce was not mad. It seems that people do indeed expose themselves to the cold temperatures of a freezing sea, in a form of cold-water immersion therapy. Bruce was doing so to help with his battle with leukaemia. He told me he had shunned conventional medicine in favour of more natural and harmonising ways of healing.

'There is no chemical being injected into this body,' he said.

Cold water was not a known cure for cancer, sadly, but it had benefits which clearly had been working for Bruce. Three times a week he would subject himself to this cold-water therapy in the North Sea.

'It helps with muscle soreness, is good for your metabolism, plus it puts me in a better mood,' he went on.

I was impressed with his resilience to the disease and his willingness to seek out alternative treatment. Some advocates also claim it can improve sleep and sharpen mental focus.

I wished Bruce all the best that day and said I hoped to see him again. After I'd told him my story, he said he would go home and promptly purchase a copy of my Everest book. I always have my sales hat with me just in case I get to wear it. You must learn to blow your own trumpet in life. No one else is going to blow it for you, and please don't quote me on that.

***

A month later, in early December, I packed up the car with towels and clean clothing. I placed my phone in a waterproof pouch and grabbed my wireless headphones. All key to my plans this morning.

I dropped the girls off at school. They were both refusing to walk the two miles to school, as it was, in Isla's words, 'Freezing cold and miserable.' Perfect, I thought.

'Come on Ella, let's go.'

My dog obediently followed, wagging her tail at the prospect of going out for a walk. I bundled her into the boot of the car, and drove to a nearby beach, five minutes from my home. The same beach where I had met Bruce. It was still early, there was hardly anyone else around. I strode down to the water's edge, placed my pack on the ground and threw a pebble for Ella. She ran off to bring it back. The game of chase and retrieve with my Labradoodle had started once again.

I stripped off to my boxer shorts, the words Comfyballs around the elasticated waist visible for anyone to see. I placed the pouch containing my phone around my neck, the headphones over my head. The hairs on my arms stood on end, goosebumps covering my body, as I tiptoed ever so slowly into the swirling icy coldness between my toes. I immediately sensed the sound of what appeared to be a screaming banshee, but realised it was me as I ran back onto the shore.

I picked up another pebble and threw it as hard as I could. Ella took off to retrieve it. This time, second time lucky, I once more made my way into the sea. On this occasion, I went further and further. The cold was overpowering. My naked exposed skin immediately began to feel numb. I was once more devoid of sensation, like that day a year ago. With Ella barking incessantly at me to get out of the water, I continued with my cold-water mission and knelt. The sea went over my shoulders. Now, I thought. With numbing fingers, I brought up a playlist of music on my phone. I found the song I was looking for.

Elbow—'One Day Like This'
I placed my headphones on, and as I had promised myself, I could not re-emerge until the song had finished. It sure was an exhilarating way to spend 6 minutes and 30 seconds.

I had gone in the sea that day not to die, but to live.

As the chorus of the song blasted out, I thought back to my time on Everest. In my head, I had always thought to myself that this would be my summit song. The song I would imagine playing out as I took my final steps on to the top of the mountain.

Stepping into a freezing cold bracing sea would have to now replace that moment in time. It was equally as fitting.

I had finally discovered who I was, and accepted my place in this crazy, chaotic and often unpredictable journey of life.

I am me, there is no one quite like me and that's the way it should be. I wouldn't want it any other way.

Right there, right then, I was the most successful I had ever been in my life. I was happy, I was content and I was living. For the first time in a long time, I felt truly alive. Freezing cold, but alive.

In the words taken from one of my favourite '80s movies:

'Life moves, pretty fast. If you don't stop and look around once in a while, you could miss it.'

Thanks, Mr Bueller, I could not have said it better myself.

ACKNOWLEDGEMENTS

Thanks to everyone who has ever inspired me, made me laugh and made me believe in myself.

Thank you to my publisher FBS Publishing for taking a chance on this book without even knowing what it was about. A great leap of faith, indeed. I hope it is rewarded.

And thanks to the editorial team for correcting my many foolish errors and mistakes.

And finally, thank you to these artists and songs for being the soundtrack to my life and for helping me out of some sticky jams more times than I care to remember. The Misadventure playlist is available from Spotify and all good record shops.

Muse—'Knights of Cydonia'
Coldplay—'Fix You'
Elbow—'One Day Like This'
Green Day—'Boulevard of Broken Dreams'
Eminem—'Lose Yourself'
Dario G—'Sunchyme'
Lucy Spraggan—'Stick the Kettle On'
Faithless— 'Insomnia'
The Verve—'Lucky Man'
Fall out Boy—'Wilson'
The Killers—'All These Things That I've Done'
David Dunn—'Today is Beautiful'

LINKS

Ellis J Stewart on Twitter @EllisJStewart

Ellis J Stewart on Instagram @ellisjstewart

Facebook Everest Dream - The Mount Everest Group
https://www.facebook.com/groups/798091403726352

FBS Publishing Ltd
www.fbs-publishing.co.uk
info@fbs-publishing.co.uk

MENTAL HEALTH USEFUL LINKS

If you or someone you know has been affected by similar issues to the ones in this book, we would like to mention the following organisations who offer non-judgemental and confidential support to anyone experiencing mental health issues.

MIND is a UK mental health charity that aims to support anyone experiencing mental health issues. They have a wide range of resources and support available. The also have advice specifically aimed at supporting people affected in whatever way by the COVID-19 pandemic.

Infoline: 0300 123 3393 9am to 6pm, Monday to Friday (except for bank holidays).
Email: info@mind.org.uk
Website: mind.org.uk

The Samaritans are a charity who offer support to anyone experiencing extreme anxiety or suicidal thoughts or simply want to talk to someone about how they are feeling.
You can get in touch with them online via chat, by telephone or email them. Their number is free to call.

24 hour telephone line: 116 123
Email: jo@samaritans.org
Website: samaritans.org
Online chat: https://webchat.samaritans.org